CONVERSATIONS WITH PLANTS

CONVERSATIONS WITH PLANTS
The Path Back to Nature

Nikki Darrell

AEON

Aeon Books Ltd
12 New College Parade
Finchley Road
London NW3 5EP

British Library Cataloguing in Publication Data

A C.I.P. for this book is available from the British Library

ISBN-13: 978-1-91159-764-3

Typeset by Medlar Publishing Solutions Pvt Ltd, India
Printed in Great Britain

www.aeonbooks.co.uk

CONTENTS

Setting some context

We have arrived in the twenty-first century with a long story of how we got here. In fact, there are many stories of how we got here since many people have been involved in the journey and its evolution up to this point. It is very important to realise that although these stories have some similarities, there are also important factors in each which we need to be informed of to get a fuller picture of the panoramic view. In the English speaking world, we often listen to a very selective version of the stories of how we got here, excluding the voices of the women, the peasants, the people of colour and other marginalised groups; it is time for us to hear some of the untold aspects the relationship between plants and people.

We can do this by reaching further into the unwritten traditions; the family and rural traditions. They are not gone; they are just not written down. And they are eroded in some places but not others.

When I did my formal training as a herbalist, there were no such things as degrees or masters in herbal medicine. I graduated the year before degrees came into being. At the same time as attending the School of Phytotherapy, I worked with a third generation herbalist, and I had also spent nearly 20 years in informal studies; each strand of learning brought its own gifts, insights and knowledge.

Although science has informed our practice beneficially in some ways, it has become a rather despotic force, rather than a tool. Academia is failing us more and more. I left the world of academia and research in the mid-1980s when Margaret Thatcher and others of the capitalist corporate model dictated that all research must have corporate funding, and yield products. Science itself has become infected by corporate capitalism and is no longer objective, neutral or impartial; it has become biased in a specific direction that is fundamentally at odds with the true nature of plant medicine.

Plants were here before people, we have co-evolved with the plants, and they collaborated with the rest of Nature in our evolution; it was the mosses that first emerged from the oceans and made air breathable for land animals and plants and started the process of creating soil. We are complex beings and so are the plants and our complexities complement each other.

Our religious culture places humans in dominion over Nature; actually, this is a false idea. Nature collaborated to evolve the human species to take care and serve and carry out a range of other ecological functions as will be elucidated during our explorations. It is a worthwhile question to meditate upon … what are the ecological functions of the human species? This shift towards dominion only happened about 10,000 years ago, a brief time span, when hierarchy and dominator models replaced the egalitarian community-based culture that was spread across the globe. Although some argue that the Golden Age never existed, there is plenty of evidence to show that it did in the times of the mound people. The political and philosophical culture of the West became one of colonialism, plunder, extraction, consumerism, technology, privilege and kyriarchy.

Previously, people worked with the plants around them. There were trade routes, exchanges of ideas and plants moved around the world with the people, joining new communities. For the ordinary people, the plants that they used were the ones that they could grow in their own area, along with small amounts of exotic spices and so forth. Most medicines were prepared at home or in local communities, and people showed a deep understanding of how to do this for the best benefit. They did not prepare many tinctures but made all manner of elegant preparations from the plants. Then the enclosures happened, and people were moved off the land and forgot those relationships. The Elite was created.

What has this all got to do with where we are today? We are at a crisis point where plant medicine holds the potential to heal many ills not just of the people but also of ecosystems and the Earth itself. But only if we remember who we are.

So, from the perspective of plants and the ordinary grassroots people there are stories that need to be heard, the stories about how people helped to create the ecosystems, working with the trees and the plants; the Kayapo, the Kogi, the walnut forests, the Amazonian forests, even the oak forests of the Western European Isles and France, the grasslands and prairies. Humans, the other animals, the plants, insects and fungi worked together. People moved freely without borders. Some settled and worked with the land around them, the land they belonged to rather than had dominion over, and they did this sustainably, not worshipping Nature but knowing they were of the natural world, not separate. The dark myth of separation has caused great wounding to the point where we have fallen into even viewing our own bodies (the piece of earth that we are) as a machine in a mechanomorphic world view overly dominated by the left neo-cortex view of the world as lifeless.

Vitality and vitalism have been written out of the current medical epistemology so that we forget that we are indeed living beings with an ability to heal ourselves and make the land around us healthy.

We are at a crucial point where we can continue to consume, pillage and plunder and view the rest of Nature as resources and commodities for us to take, or we can come back to our senses, slow down and realise that we are at present on a pathological path that will lead to declining health for ourselves and our kin before we extinct ourselves; we can come back to ourselves and remember how to make it beautiful. We can return to sanity and clarity.

> It's time to snatch our futures back from the experts. Time to ask, in ordinary language, the public question, and to demand, in ordinary language, the public answer.
>
> Arundhati Roy (The End of Imagination, p. 188)

We need to move from dominator models to community and partnership, letting go of privilege and entitlement and seeing that there is an elegant sufficiency for all and that there are much healthier possibilities.

I came to the vocation of being a plant medicine person because the plants called me. The plants are so incredibly generous and provide so much for us. They have been objectified for hundreds of years, and it is wonderful to now see science validating what authentic people have always known—plants are sentient and conscious. They are intelligent and hold great wisdom. We are not the only species with consciousness, morality, intelligence and the ability to communicate. So now it is time to listen to the green ones and work with them, to become biocentric, ecocentric and nurture the biophilia we are born with, to engender biognosis and learn what we really were evolved to be; not rapists and vandals but in service to our community.

PART I

OUR GREEN ALLIES

This part of the book focuses on the plants in regard to their anatomy and how different parts act as medicines; plant families and their therapeutic properties; plant constituents and our ability to sense the constituents and brief ideas on actions; evolving ways of working with them to improve biodiversity, ecosystem health and the concept of wild gardening.

CHAPTER ONE

Understanding plant anatomy, their parts and their medicine

All life is descended from a common ancestry, so there are many similarities between plants and people, especially when we look at a cellular level. Both have cells that contain a nucleus, mitochondria, endoplasmic reticulum, cytoplasm and have a cell membrane.

Mitochondria are now thought to have originally been separate organisms that negotiated a synergistic relationship with a eukaryotic host. My daughter insists that I tell the story like this: Once upon a time in the primordial soup there were all sorts of little beings (bacteria, our common ancestors) floating around. Some had a good tough cell membrane which meant they had good boundaries; some were really good at producing energy from food taken in and making it into ATP; others could capture the energy of sunlight and produce their own food. One day, one with a tough coating and one who was good at producing ATP bumped into one another, and they fell to talking; after a while, they realised they each had something to offer each other and the tough one agreed to let the energy one in through the boundary, offering protection in exchange for energy production; and so mitochondria came into being. And then some of these symbiotic ecosystem cells decided to negotiate with the ones who could photosynthesise and let them in because that meant they no longer had to waste so much time and energy wandering around looking for food, they could just do it with the aid of the chloroplasts.

It is also interesting to note that the DNA of the main cells is inherited in equal part from the male and female parent (the pollen and ovum in the case of the plant, or the sperm and egg in the case of animals). However, both mitochondria and chloroplasts come solely from the maternal line as part of the matter of the egg or ovum.

Then there are important differences between plant and animal cells. In plants cells the following structures are present:

- The cell membrane is surrounded by a rigid non-living cell wall in order to give structure and form to the plant as it has no skeleton. When the cell wall is removed, the cell is known as a protoplast.
- Vacuoles are present in plant cells. In most mature plant cells, there is a single large vacuole that takes up most of the cell's volume. The vacuole is contained within a membrane called a tonoplast and is filled with an aqueous solution in which many substances are dissolved. The function of the vacuole is to act as a recycling reservoir for certain substances and a waste storage area for others. It also exerts pressure against the cell wall to maintain turgidity or rigidity in the non-lignified areas of the plant. When a plant experiences water stress, it loses water from the vacuole, the pressure drops, and this leads to wilting which reduces the area of water loss and therefore protects the plant from further stress.
- Plant cells also contain chloroplasts, organelles containing chloro-phyll, the green pigment which traps the energy from sunlight to allow the plant to manufacture its own food. The plant can use sun-light, carbon dioxide and water to manufacture sugars, and recycle oxygen. Thus, plants are necessary for the recycling of oxygen, and are the only organisms which can create food. Animals must either eat plants or other animals. Other plastids may be present, which are organelles that store pigment (chromoplast) or starch (amyloplast). In common with mitochondria, chloroplasts contain their own DNA and ribosomes of a form similar to prokaryotes and have also been hypothesised to have originally been symbiotic prokaryotes.
- Plant cell walls also have a middle lamella containing pectin.
- There are plasmodesmata or pores in the cell membrane.

Plant structure and anatomy

We will focus on the structure and form of seed-forming green plants (Spermatophyta) since these are the majority of plants that we prepare medicines from.

The main structures of the plant are the roots, stems, leaves, flowers and fruits; also, the meristem tissues which are analogous to stem cells. Each structure is modified to suit the particular environment of the plant. In general terms, the plant's structure is organised from a single main axis, divided into the root system beneath the ground and the shoot system above the ground.

Meristematic tissue

Meristematic tissue is capable of dividing to produce new cells to allow growth to continue. When meristematic regions are active, they produce undifferentiated cells, some of which stay undifferentiated to maintain the meristem regions and others enter into differentiation to form the necessary plant tissues. There are several types, according to where in the plant they occur:

- Apical at the tip of the plant
- Marginal around the leaf margin
- Lateral to allow an increase in stem and root girth in perennials
- Intercalary, above the younger nodes of monocotyledon stems, e.g. bamboo
- Basal meristems at the base of some monocotyledonous leaves

There are three layers to the meristematic tissue—the protoderm (forms epidermis), procambium (forms xylem and phloem), ground meristem (forms cortex and pith). Also, the cork cambium forms bark.

Meristematic tissues and sprouted seeds are full of beneficial enzymes, plant growth factors and other components which help with tissue repair. The plant growth factor kinetin has been shown to repair skin and also to help prevent nervous tissue degeneration in diseases like Parkinson's which means that eating sprouted seeds, microgreens and young spring leaves is highly beneficial for our health. Microgreens have been shown to be 4–10 times more nutrient dense than mature vegetables.

Roots

Roots are normally underground, although some plants evolved to grow in environments where there is a lot of moisture in the air and therefore have aerial roots as well. The functions of the roots are to absorb water and nutrients; to serve as an anchor; to store nutrients; to help communication within the soil by releasing various compounds and sensing those from other organisms and interacting with the mycorrhiza; they also host some commensiles such as the nitrogen-fixing bacteria that reside in the nodules of leguminous roots. The roots normally grow down into the soil due to the influence of amyloplasts—plastids containing starch granules that respond to gravity (geotropism). The direction of growth is also influenced by water sources (hydrotropism) and nutrient sources (chemotropism), obstacles such as stones and by secretions from the roots of surrounding plants that sometimes act as repellents. The tip of the root is protected by the root cap; the golgi bodies of the root cap produce a mucilage to ease the movement of the roots through the soil. Roots also have an outer layer of parenchymal cells for storing food. There is a band of cells or pericycle from which new roots grow.

Roots may be modified to act as storage organs for carbohydrates over winter; tap roots and tubers. They may store other compounds such as essential oils.

Roots can differ radically in shape and form, depending on the type of plant. Roots have an immense surface area and communicate with mycorrhizal mats within the soil, as well as bacteria (including the nitrogen-fixing bacteria that live in symbiotic nodules on the roots of leguminous plants) and communicate with other plants by releasing various chemicals into the soil. Roots also 'read' the soil: the information and chemical meaning released by the breakdown of dead plant and animal material, by the excrement of animals and the soil's microflora and adjust their physiology accordingly to bring more balance to the ecosystem.

Root medicines tend to be nutritive tonics. The polysaccharides that they contain are valuable immune modulants. Some roots contain essential oils which are good nerve tonics and may also be antimicrobial (*Inula, Rubus fructicosus*). Many roots are adaptogen tonics, helping us to deal better with stress of all kinds. Many roots are also foods. Since the harvest of roots can mean that the plant is no longer able to grow, we need to be discerning in our use of these medicines. However, roots such as *Inula, Echinacea, Armoracia* can be harvested and propagated from root cuttings at the same time. *Angelica* harvest is a destructive one, taking the whole root.

Stems

Stems are normally above the ground, and their functions are to support other structures (leaves, tendrils, reproductive organs) and to carry water and nutrients up through the plant, and to carry sugars, waste products and other metabolites from the leaves down through the plant. The stem is divided into internodes (the spaces between the points where lateral stems, leaves or flowers arise) and nodes (the places where these structures arise). Modifications include bulbs, corms, turions, runners, stolons, rhizomes, stem tubers, droppers, bulbils, thorns, tendrils, suckers and offsets. Rhizomes are specialised stems that run under the ground; normally used for vegetative reproduction and for storage. Tubers are specialised root or stem tissue used as storage organs. Corms are specialised stems. In woody plants, the stem, and sometimes the roots, are covered with a hardened protective material called bark. Bark is laid down over structures that are older than a year.

Vascular plants contain bundles of vessels (vascular bundles) to transport water, nutrients and metabolites through the plant. There are two types, xylem and phloem, which are both produced from the cambium. Xylem carries water and nutrients up from the roots to the rest of the plant, whilst phloem carries metabolites such as sugars and waste products away from the leaves; although this is a simplification. Dicotyledonous (those with two baby leaves in the seed) plants have a ring of vascular bundles. Monocotyledonous plants (those with one baby leaf in the seed, mainly grasses and similar plants such as maize) have scattered vascular bundles.

The stem is covered by the epidermis. In woody plants, there is a layer of cork and/or bark under this. There are other layers that make up the cortex, and beneath this lies the endodermis. Within the endodermis lies the medulla, which is made up of parenchyma through which the vascular tissues run. Cork and bark serve as strengthening tissues. At the core is the heartwood; this contains dead xylem, vascular cambium and sapwood with living xylem. Annular rings are formed by the fact that stems contain about ten times more xylem than phloem.

Soluble materials such as food produced in the leaves, dissolved salts absorbed from the soil and growth substances manufactured in the plant are moved in the vascular tissue by a process known as translocation. The pith of the stem is a local food store. Barks contain lignin and tannins to protect the inner structures, and they are useful astringents that can help to tighten tissues and drive out moisture as well as helping to heal damage tissues and reduce haemorrhage. Some also contain essential oils that are often protective against microbial invasion (for example, cinnamon).

Leaves

Leaves absorb sunlight to enable photosynthesis to occur, provide a large enough area for transpiration (the excretion of water), and to allow rapid gaseous exchange between the cells and their external environment to facilitate photosynthesis. They can also be used to store food and water. There may be modified leaves that are adapted to perform other functions. The structure of the leaf can vary markedly depending on the plants' environment.

Leaves contain protein, vitamins, minerals and may contain essential oils and other constituents. Many wild food leaves contain appreciable levels of protein (for example, nettle and plantain).

Flowers

Plants bearing true flowers are known as angiosperms and have fruit contained in a fleshy carpellary covering. The ways in which flowers occur and are arranged on the plant are constant for a species, but they are very variable throughout the world of angiosperms. There is great variation in shape, form, number of petals, colour, aroma and the arrangement of the flowers (the inflorescence).

Some plants have separate male and female flowers (maize), whilst others take it to the extreme of only bearing female or male flowers on an individual plant, e.g., holly, juniper, yew, nettle. In such cases, two plants, one of each gender, are needed to produce fruit. Plants with male and female flowers on separate plants are called dioecious, and those with single-sex flowers, but both male and female on the same plant are monoecious. These adaptations help to ensure that plants do not self-fertilise, ensuring greater genetic diversity and therefore the ability to adapt to a wider variety of niches and habitats.

Flowers are made up of various parts:

The pedicel (flower stem) gives rise to the receptacle.

Sepals (collectively the calyx) and petals are similar to leaves but simpler in structure. They contain chloroplasts and chromoplasts that contain other pigments. The petals and sepals together form the outer protective layer around the sex organs known as the perianth. Sepals protect the bud and peel back when the flower opens. Petals attract and guide pollinators towards the sex organs.

Stamen is the term for the male organs. The anthers produce pollen grains—the male sex cells which are analogous to sperm; the anther is supported by a filament. The male parts are collectively known as the androecium.

The carpel and gynaecium are the female parts. The lower part of the carpel is differentiated into the ovule-containing ovary. The upper part is the style, and the terminal platform is called the stigmatic surface or a pistil on which the pollen falls. Nectaries are specialised glands found in the flower, for the purpose of attracting insect and animal pollinators. We will not discuss the minutiae of pollination, the ability or inability of different species to self-pollinate and so on here. Suffice to say that pollination involves the transfer of pollen from the anthers to the style. Some plants can be pollinated by their own flowers; other plants require another member of their species to produce a viable seed. Pollen transfer may occur by wind, bees and other insects, birds, small mammals such as bats or by plain gravity. When the pollen lands on the style it exudes certain enzymes that allow it to bore a tunnel down the style to the ovum/ova in order to fertilise them. The seed embryo has a small chain of connecting cells that attach it to the mother (suspensor cells); some inter-species incompatibility is due to the inability to produce viable suspensor cells. Such embryos can be excised and cultured in tissue culture environments to allow development of an embryo—plant in vitro fertilisation, cloning, test tube babies.

Flowers contain pigments (many of which are bitter) which often have antioxidant properties that help with tissue repair and reducing inflammation. Flowers often contain essential oils which are beneficial nervines and which have antiseptic properties. Many flowers are excellent nervines. They also nourish our sense of beauty visually and by their aromas.

Seeds and fruit

The seed consists of the embryo and the testa or seed coat, which encloses and protects the embryo and has a small pore or micropyle that allows gaseous and water exchange and the hilum which is the scar where it was attached to the ovary. There may also be a mass of food storing tissue within the testa called the endosperm. Some fruits have a fleshy layer or pericarp which protects the seeds. It consists of the exocarp, mesocarp and endocarp.

Seeds are full of protein, starches, essential fatty acids, minerals and vitamins that the plant embryo needs to germinate and grow. Many of our wild seeds are as nourishing as some of the more widely sold ones. Plantain seed was traditionally used in a similar way to psyllium and added to bread and baking. Nettle seed contains a wide range of essential fatty acids and proteins and is a traditional winter energy food; it can be dried and added to baking or preserved in oil or vinegar.

Fruits contain acids, sugars, vitamins, minerals and soft fibre. They are also nutritive tonics. The pigments they contain are often anthocyanins which are particularly beneficial for repairing the blood vessels, reducing inflammation and promoting nerve repair.

CHAPTER TWO

Plants as alchemists (including organoleptic exercises)

Plants are amazing chemists, producing a multitude of constituents using various pathways to synthesise them, and this is a huge area of learning in itself, not within the remit of this book but worth exploring to help one realise just how talented they are.

We are going to focus on some of these groups of constituents, their therapeutic actions in the human (as well as their value to the plant) and how we can use our senses to appreciate them and to recognise the plant's qualities and attributes. Indeed, our senses (once trained) are better at this task than any machine.

We need to engage as many senses as possible in order to truly listen to our plant allies and our patients, and to be holistic in our assessment of them. We have tended to become extremely reductionist in our relationship with our plant allies, relying on analytical facts, labelling, putting in boxes rather than remembering that they are living sentient beings who share their meanings with us, who are healers in their own right and that our role is to listen to the people and listen to the plants; our skill is in knowing them well enough that we can see which plant will help re-align the person at that particular time into a healing balance.

Each plant contains many different constituents which may seem to have conflicting actions to our surface analytical minds (the same way that many of the people we know have different aspects to their personalities). Different aspects are more accessible to different people, depending on our sensory perception; each of us is likely to read the medicine of the plant somewhat differently. However, we can work with our sensory acuity to develop the skill of sensing out the different meanings and getting a whole feeling of the plant's persona; seeing, feeling, hearing, tasting, smelling out all the different parts that make up the whole. From there we can understand that the appropriate part of the plant will feed into a person when that medicine is needed; that this may vary from time to time and that what seems to be present only in tiny amounts might actually make up a major part of the medicine that the plant feeds into the world.

We will explore some of the major groups of plant constituents (real-ising that some are classified under more than one category; this is just an introduction into honing these skills, which can be a lifetime's work) and how to use our senses to feel what is there. Indigenous healers never had analytical laboratories to enable them to stick labels on the molecules within the plant, but they used their senses to identify the meanings. It may be a far more accurate way of doing it; tuning in with all our brains and our senses. The mistake that was made with kava did not happen using such an approach; it happened when such things were rejected, and laboratory techniques and machines were relied upon (machines and laboratory techniques can be very valuable but not at the expense of our common senses).

First a note or two on the senses, the study of which could take an entire book or library.

Olfaction

We smell through the left and right nostrils separately. Olfactory nerves are directly connected to the same side of the brain as the stimulus, and there are no synaptic junctions between the nerves and the brain. When aroma molecules are present in the air, we do not need to consciously perceive them in order to be affected by them. Sometimes molecules are present in parts per billion, and they affect us; whereas, they have to be present at parts per million in order for us to perceive them.

We do not have to be familiar with a smell in order to elicit a response. The smell of chocolate will encourage a baby of 11 weeks to produce 'happy brain waves' and increased digestive secretions. Olfaction is a precognitive event to language; a metanym is a nonverbal communication, whilst metaphors are linguistic, and a metanymic association occurs in a baby recognising its mother's breast milk long before they can make metaphorical connections.

We do not have to be consciously aware of an aroma for it to affect our mood. People's perception of smell varies as much as their perception of sound and visual stimuli; thus, what one person appreciates may not appeal to another. People can also have blind spots in their repertoire of aromas; these are known as specific anosmias, where people are unable to detect certain aromas. There are also some unfortunate individuals that perceive all odours as fetid and unpleasant. This has a strong influence on their appetite. It is possible to educate one's nose to be able to pick up a wider range of aromas. The easiest aromas to decipher are those of the citrus family (they are monoterpene based and therefore they are small, simple molecules). However, perfumiers spend many years training their noses and building up a bank of fragrance memories which enable them to create blends on paper.

The nose is the organ of olfaction, and the olfactory cells are positioned at the top of the nose. This is why the deep sniff is the preferred method of getting a true odour.

The olfactory bulb also connects closely with the hypothalamus. Smell could therefore influence many of our bodily processes. There are amazing implications as to how this could initiate 'trickle down' effects on an emotional and physical level.

Our sense of smell tires easily. If we smell many odours in quick succession, our nose gives up and loses the ability to detect anything. When smelling samples and medicines to assess qualities, it is therefore important to take breaks.

One interesting fact is that we need a familiar smell environment in order to feel happy. One other interesting vignette is that odour has not always been so neglected by medicine. The Greeks believed that various aromas had certain healing properties (the scent of apples was good for headache and migraine; narcissi were a strong narcotic). Doctors also used to use smell in a different way. The odour of the patient was used in diagnosis; infections such as the plague and typhoid gave the patient a particular body odour.

Olfaction and chemoreception

We perceive smell via the first cranial nerve or olfactory nerve; however, there are other structures involved. The trigeminal nerve is involved in some smell and taste experiences. For example, with black pepper or chilli, a branch of the trigeminal nerve is irritated, adding to the spiciness of the taste and smell, whilst with menthol-containing tastes and odours the nerve is refrigerated which adds to the cool fresh taste and smell of peppermint. Since the trigeminal nerve extensively enervates the face, this explains how some aromas seem to affect the whole face. There are two other structures that are involved in some species: the septal organ and the vomer-nasal or Jacobson's organ. This is what a snake or a cat is using when it opens its mouth widely in a seeming yawn, whilst in fact smelling the air—Flaymsan's response. It is also active from about the fifth month in the womb in humans, allowing the baby to 'smell' the amniotic fluid. It was thought that it turned off at birth; however, more recent work suggests it stays active in many people, giving them a rather different perception of smell. It takes us longer to name smells than colours or sounds.

We can divide odour compounds into families of similar aromas or similar chemical structures. It is likely that there are different types of olfactory receptor cells which pick up the different odour groups and it is possible that their activity can increase and that we can learn to tune this sense.

For any aroma there is a detection threshold and a higher recognition threshold; at the lower level, we know we are smelling something but there needs to be a sufficient quantity of molecules present for us to recognise what we are smelling; training and practice can definitely hone the ability to recognise at a lower level and definitively differentiate between similar smells.

Touch

The mouth is full of sensory receptors; some of what we think of as taste is actually stimulation of the trigeminal nerve (cooling effect of menthol, spicy burning of cayenne, mucilage's soothing effect). Children put stuff in their mouths when they start to explore the world; it is natural to use the mouth for touch exploration as well as taste and smell. There are various sensations we can detect with touch such as heat, cold, tickle, light touch, prickle, pain, smoothness, roughness. We can also use our hands to touch the plants, to feel their textures.

Taste

There are five primary tastes sweet, sour, salty, bitter, umami (a savoury taste which is our ability to sense B vitamins in foods such as yeast and meat); we also have taste receptors for fatty acids and calcium and pungent (which is really a touch sensation). Our taste receptors are not just in our mouths. They are located throughout the digestive system and in other regions of the body. Their location means that certain tastes can provoke reflex actions in the body or have a particular therapeutic effect. We have sour receptors along our spine, and when we taste something sour we initially tense then relax. We have sweet receptors in our kidney-adrenal complex, and therefore we give warm, sweet drinks when someone is feeling stressed or shocked. We have bitter tastes in a number of different areas, so these do not just work on the liver and digestion, they also help to promote the peripheral circulation and have effects on the lungs and sinuses amongst other tissues. In various traditional medicine systems, each taste is considered as relating to a particular element and therefore to specific emotions and types of people. In Traditional Chinese Medicine, bitter is considered as relating to fire and therefore to joy/ecstasy; sour relates to wood and therefore to the liver and anger; salty relates to water, the kidney/bladder energy and fear; pungent corresponds to the metal element, the lungs and large intestine and the emotion of grief; sweet relates to the earth, the energy of the stomach and spleen and therefore to worry.

In addition to this, some of what we think of as taste is actually to do with what we sense with smell or with touch (the texture in our mouths).

This is a simplified version but can give some interesting ideas about linking taste to the energetic medicine of a plant. However, the important thing is to tune in and listen to what the plant is telling you.

Sound

We can certainly listen with our inner ears and pick up all sorts of information that the plants are giving us, and there is more about this below when we talk about feeling perception. However, we can also listen to the sounds that plants make in regard to the noises they make when the wind blows through them. Try listening to a pine forest and the way it sounds so similar to the waves and the ocean; both are known to release large quantities of negative ions which are really beneficial for our health. Other plants make sounds when releasing their seeds explosively.

Sight

When working with plants, we look with both the ordinary eyes and the inner eyes. With the ordinary eyes we may take note of the fact that a plant is particularly succulent like aloe vera, and is likely to contain a soothing mucilage; we may note that fruits are deep red or purple and therefore are likely to contain large amounts of anthocyanins; we can note the form of a plant and deduce which botanical family it belongs to. With the inner eyes we may reach further into these perceptions and see that *Acanthus* flower stems look like the spinal column (it is used to correct subluxations of the skeletal system), and that dulse is a deep red (it contains high levels of vitamin B_{12}, needed to build healthy red blood cells). Angelica leaves are reminiscent of large open lungs, whilst the stem has red streaks showing its benefits for the circulation, and the flower/seed heads look like a halo reminding us that it is wonderful for calming the mind. Rheum has bright red stems denoting its benefits as a blood purifier, whilst its rootstock looks like the plant would certainly move constipation (it looks like an extremely large, dark turd). The list is endless. This is analogous to the old Doctrine of Signatures, but we can really take ownership of our own ability to make these connections. When we are using our sight, we can ask questions like what draws us? Do we prefer certain colours, textures, shapes or is it that the plant reminds us of something?

Synaesthesia

Some people are synaesthetic, possibly as many as 1 in 23. This means that they experience a cross over between their sensory modalities so that smells may have colours or sounds and so forth. The condition may be due to the dominance of the limbic system; it can lead to a certain amount of defensiveness due to difficulty in communicating in the civilised world. Some researchers posit the possibility that synaesthesia is actually our natural way of being.

Feeling perception

Feeling perception is not in the conventional list of senses but is a most valuable one when engaged in this work; sometimes when we engage our senses working with a plant or examining its medicine, we find that information comes from another sense—the heart perception. We get a sense of emotional tone since the heart is the organ of emotional perception and our emotional memories. The impressions we receive through our heart perception may be more of a gestalt rather than a left-brain style lecture on therapeutics from the plant (although the information does sometimes arrive in that form). As we receive impressions, emotions or memories, or impressions of animals, colours, or whatever arrives, it is good to note these down and see what they signify to you. We can also feel where the plant's energy, its medicine, enters our body and where it moves to.

One day we were sitting with a group of students, encouraging them to participate in trying to sense into the *Kalanchoe pinnata* (also known as miracle leaf or love plant) plants around the room; when I asked for feedback one of the students said that what came into her head was walking in the forest of her native Lithuania when she was younger; this plant really brings us home to our heart and the feeling of being safe and loved and nurtured. Another student came in from sitting with a myrtle plant. When she started talking her voice took on the gentleness of someone talking to a small infant, that soft tone, her arms moved into a loving cuddle. She was expressing the gestalt of how myrtle is used for small children and babies, especially to help them with respiratory and urinary infections. It is also traditionally included in bridal bouquets to symbolise ...

Gut instinct

Gut instinct and the gut-brain will be discussed in more detail later on. Suffice to say that as soon as we take a plant medicine into our mouth messages are sent to our gut-brain via the vagus nerve, touch receptors in the mouth and the taste receptors to tell us about it. As it moves through our digestive tract, we receive more and more information via our gut-brain, from our microflora. Our gut-brain is truly about reading the meanings from our food and our instincts learning about our environment this way. Learning about our medicines this way.

Common sense

Using our common sense is key in our explorations. For example, if it does not look right, smell right or feel right do not taste it ...

Finally, when we take in our medicine it is better if the substance is spaced out in a similar way to how it is in the living plant; grazing on fresh herbs is a glorious way to learn from them. If you are using dried herbs, a tea is better than just chewing the dried plant since it spaces out the information, makes it easier to read. Similarly, if you are working with tinctures, it is better to dilute them in a little water, partly so that the tastes are not overwhelmed by the alcohol but also to spread out the information so that you can discern the whole story.

Organoleptic exercises

Here are some examples of constituents and their actions and what effect they may have on one's senses. These are just a starting point to encourage one into further exploration.

Mucilages and gums

Mucilages feel slimy, like jelly. Gums feel sticky.

These are polysaccharides or glycans, which are high molecular weight polymers of sugars. They are water-soluble but do not dissolve in alcohol so are best used by infusion or decoction. They have a demulcent action internally and an emollient action externally; they are soothing and protecting to irritated tissues. When a demulcent is taken internally, it soothes the lining of the gastrointestinal tract (GIT), and this triggers a reflex action in the linings of the other organs. Gums and mucilages are also useful as bulk laxatives and can also relieve diarrhoea by soothing the mucosa.

Examples of plants containing mucilages and gums are: pectin in stewed apple, *Ulmus falva*, *Plantago* species, *Tussilago farfara*, *Verbascum thapsus*, *Althea officinalis*, *Symphytum officinalis*, *Chondrus crispus* (and other seaweeds), *Cetraria* (and other lichens), *Acacia sp.*

Some polysaccharides have an immuno-stimulating effect.

Inulin and fructans help to stabilise blood sugar and have diuretic and immunostimulating effects. They are found in *Inula helenium*,

Arctium lappa, Cyanara scolymus, Cichorium intybus, Taraxacum officinale, Echinacea spp., Helianthus sp.

Phenols

Phenols tend to give a hot or drying sensation in the mouth and can feel irritating.

These are one of the largest groups of plant secondary metabolites. They are molecules which have at least one hydroxyl group attached to a benzene ring. They may also have other groups, such as methyl groups. Simple phenols consist of a benzene ring with one hydrogen replaced by a hydroxyl group. They are found in many different classes and species of plants. They are tertiary alcohols which act like acids.

They are bactericidal, antiseptic and anthelmintic. In correct doses, they are anti-inflammatory internally. Externally, they are irritating to the skin and mucous membranes.

Examples are:

- Salicylic acid found in *Filipendula ulmaria, Salix alba, Gaultheria procumbens, Betula sp., Viburnum opulus*
- Thymol found in *Thymus vulgaris*
- Eugenol found in *Eugenia caryophyllum*

Other phenylpropanoid molecules include:

- Cynarin found in *Cyanara scolymus*—hepatoprotective and hypocholesterolaemic
- Curcumin, a yellow pigment in *Curcuma longa*, which is a significant anti-inflammatory, hypotensive and hepatoprotective
- Arbutin in leaves of *Pyrus communis* and *Arctostaphylos uva-ursi*—a urinary tract antiseptic and diuretic

Lignans

Lignans are found in grains and pulses and have phytoestrogenic effects.

Other lignans are schizandrins found in *Schizandra chinensis* which reverse the destruction of liver cells by induction of cytochrome P-450.

Flavonolignans from *Silybum marianum* (also classed as flavonoids) are also hepatoprotective.

Tannins

These are extremely astringing and drying and are polyphenols. They occur in tree bark, insect galls, leaves, stems and fruit. They are non-crystalline and give a mild acid when dissolved in water. They are strongly astringent e.g. *Camellia sinensis*. They precipitate proteins and are therefore used to produce leather from animal hides.

There are two types:

- Hydrolysable tannins which hydrolyse to give gallic acid and glucose. They dissolve in both water and alcohol readily, e.g., *Geranium maculatum*, *Agrimonia eupatoria*, *Arctostaphylos uva-ursi*, *Rubus idaeus*, *Geum urbanum*, *Quercus robur*, *Potentilla erecta*, *Achillea millefoliun*.
- Condensed tannins yield phlobaphenes, which are insoluble red residues, upon hydrolysis. They are only partially soluble in water and alcohol, but glycerine improves solubility.

As astringents, tannins cause contraction of tissues, blanching and wrinkling of mucous membranes and reduced exudation. As they precipitate proteins and polysaccharides, their application to the skin causes hardening of the epidermis, reduced absorption and protection against irritation. They also have an antimicrobial action, and many constrict blood vessels so reducing bleeding.

Other actions include:

- Protection of inflamed mucous membranes
- Reduction of hypersecretion
- Reduction of inflammation and swelling with infection
- Haemostatic with small wounds
- Reduction of uterine bleeding
- Binding effect in the gut

Pro-anthocyanidins or pycnogenols are condensed tannins derived from pine bark and grape seeds which are potent antioxidants for the vascular system. Similar compounds are found in *Crataegus sp.*

Condensed tannins are found in tea and red wine. Green tea is especially rich in epigallocatechins.

Tannins can lead to the reduced absorption of proteins, iron and other nutrients and therefore should not be consumed with food. It is also a consideration when formulating herbal medicines.

Coumarins

Coumarins smell like freshly mown grass or hay.

These are found in a wide range of plant species and have diverse actions. They often occur as glucosides.

- Aesculin in *Aesculus hippocanastum.*
- *Melilotus officinalis* contains coumarins which metabolise to dicoumarol which act as an anticoagulant.
- Bergapten (a furanocoumarin) *Apium graveolens* and *Citrus bergamia* photosensitise the skin.
- Psoralen from *Ammi majus* has been used to treat vitiligo and psoriasis in conjunction with sunlight but can lead to burns.
- Khellin in *Ammi visnaga* is a powerful, smooth muscle relaxant, used to treat high blood pressure and asthma.

Flavonoids

Flavonoids are bitter. They are white and yellow pigments.

They are anti-inflammatory and help to maintain healthy circulation. Rutin found in buckwheat *Fagopyrum esculentum*, lemon pith and hesperidin strengthens capillary walls.

Flavonoids also assist in the absorption and utilisation of vitamin C. They have an action of protecting against environmental stress by stabilising membranes and antioxidant effects.

- Baicalein in *Scutellaria baicalensis* inhibits pro-inflammatory metabolites such as prostaglandins and leukotrienes.
- Quercetin and others are effective inhibitors of the release of histamine. They inhibit a number of stages of inflammation including granulation tissue formation.
- Rutin will reduce oedema in corneal and conjunctival tissue and will decrease capillary permeability, helping with diabetes, chronic

venous insufficiency, haemorrhoids, scurvy, varicose ulcers, and bruising.

- Silymarin, in *Carduus marianus*, quercetin and taxifolin all protect liver mitochondria and microsomes from lipid peroxidation.
- Isoflavones are flavonoid isomers which occur on the Leguminosae, including all beans and pulses, *Glycyrrhiza glabra*, *Medicago sativa* and *Trifolium pratense*. They are phyto-oestrogens which help protect against breast cancer, probably other cancers, and can help reduce symptoms of PMS and menopause.

Anthocyanins

Anthocyanins are red, purple or blue.

These are condensed tannins found in red, blue and black fruits which are the pigments which give them their colour. *Ribes*, *Rubus* and *Vaccinium* fruits all show superoxide radical scavenging and antilipo-peroxidant activities; in other words, they are antioxidants.

Volatile oils

Volatile Oils have a wide range of aromas.

Although volatile oils generally only make up less than 1% of the plant, they are so strong in their therapeutic action that they are still significant in herbal/galenic preparations. They are also distilled to prepare essential oils. Many oils contain over 50 constituents of various chemical structures:

- Hydrocarbons/terpenes, containing only carbon and hydrogen
- Alcohols—generally antimicrobial and immunostimulating and tonic *(reminiscent of ethanol, in other words vodka or other spirits)*
- Aldehydes—sedative, antiviral and antimicrobial *(lemon sherbert)*
- Aromatic aldehydes (spicy and warming)
- Ketones—mucolytic, cicatrisant. Some are neurotoxic and abortifacient in high dose *(soft powdery aroma)*
- Phenols—strongly antimicrobial, dermal and mucous membrane irritants *(hot penetrating aroma)*
- Phenyl methyl ethers/phenolic ethers *(Aniseed/liquorice aroma)*
- Oxides—expectorant and mucolytic *(like Eucalyptus)*

- Esters—sedative and antispasmodic (*sweet, soft, soothing aroma with the exception of methyl salicylate which is the characteristic odour of wintergreen*)
- Acids—soothing to the skin (*vinegary*)

Others include allyl isothiocyanate, discussed under glucosilinates, and allyl sulphides found in the Allium family.

Essential oils studies and aromatherapy are a very broad subject, deserving of more space. Some important herbs containing volatile oils are: *Melaleuca alternifolia, Rosmarinus officinalis, Thymus vulgaris, Matricaria recutita, Salvia officinalis, Cinnamomum zeylanicum, Syzgium aromaticum, Zingiber officinalis, Origanum marjoranum, Origanum vulgare, Lavandula officinalis, Foeniculum vulgare, Mentha x piperita, Anethum graveolens.*

Saponins

Saponins taste and feel soapy.

They are glycosides whose active moieties are soluble in water and produce a lather. They lower surface tension, producing a soap like an effect on membranes and the skin. These are divided into two classes—steroidal and triterpenoid. As steroidal saponins have a similar structure to steroidal hormones in the body, they often have a hormonal type effect, e.g., *Glycyrrhiza glabra, Dioscorea villosa.* Triterpenoid saponins are often expectorants acting via stimulation of a reflex in the upper digestive tract. e.g., *Primula veris, Verbascum thapsus, Viola tricolor et odorata, Bellis perennis.* Because saponins increase the permeability of membranes, they should be used cautiously topically, and never on broken skin since their introduction into the bloodstream can cause lysis of red blood cells. This effect is nullified by digestion.

Bitters

Bitters are characterised by their taste rather than their chemical structure and cover a range of different molecules including iridoids, monoterpenes and others. The bitter taste stimulates the secretion of saliva and secretion from other digestive organs. This can lead to a dramatic increase in appetite and improvement of digestive function. They are normally taken 10–15 minutes before eating. They are traditionally used to improve liver function and overall digestive function, as well as draining trapped heat and moving the circulation. Herbs that contain bitters include *Gentiana lutea, Taraxacum officinale radix, Artemisia absinthium, Carduus marianum, Humulus lupulus, Valeriana officinalis, Marrubium vulgare, Menyanthes trifoliata, Harpagophytum procumbens.*

Alkaloids

A large and diverse group of compounds which are not always easy to classify. They often have dramatic therapeutic effects, particularly on the nervous system. examples are:

- Ephedrine raises blood pressure and classed as a protoalkaloid
- Pyridine-piperidine alkaloids, e.g., nicotine, lobeline
- Quinoline alkaloids—quinine from *Cinchona sp.*
- Isoquinoline alkaloids which include morphine, berberine, hydrastine
- Tropane alkaloids include atropine, hyoscyamine, scopolamine
- Quinolizidine alkaloids—sparteine
- Pyrrolizidine alkaloids
- Indole alkaloids reserpine, vinblastine, vincristine

Minerals

Taste salty or chalky.
   Many medicinal plants and food plants are rich in various minerals. *Equisetum arvense* is rich in silica; *Taraxacum officinale* leaf is rich in potassium and many others besides.

Glycosides

Glycosides are molecules which consist of a sugar moiety attached to one or more non-sugar moiety; they are hydrolysed by enzymes or acids into a glycone (sugar) and an aglycone—the active portion, which may be a phenol, alcohol or sulphur compound. Many are toxic in overdose, especially cyanogenic and cardiac glycosides, but cooking generally deactivates them.

Cardiac glycosides

The aglycone is a steroidal compound. These compounds have a strong direct action on the cardiac muscle which can help to support its strength and rate of contraction when it is failing. They are also significantly diuretic, and by this mechanism can reduce the blood pressure. However, they increase atrial and ventricular myocardial excitability and can lead to arrhythmias. They also decrease the rate of atrioventricular conduction, increase vagal tone and myocardial sensitivity to vagal impulses.

The stronger of these drugs are prescription only, e.g. digotoxin from *Digitalis purpurea*, digoxin from *Digitalis lanata*, *Convallaria majalis* (convallotoxin, convalloside), *Urginea maritima*.

Cyanogenic glycosides

Cyanogenic Glycosides smell and taste of bitter almonds.

They contain nitrogen in the form of hydrocyanic or prussic acid. Examples are amygdalin and prunasin found in members of the Rosaceae, particularly the *Prunus* genus. They are used in low doses for their expectorant, sedative and digestive action; also relaxant for the heart and muscles, e.g., *Prunus serotina* which contains prunasin and is used as a cough remedy. *Sambucus nigra* fruits or elderberries also contain cyanogenic glycosides.

Glucosilonates

Taste and smell of mustard/cabbage, pungent and sulphurous.

Glucosilonates are found mainly in the Brassicaceae, although similar compounds are found in the *Alliums*. They are formed by the decarboxylation of amino acids such as tyrosine, phenylalanine and tryptophan. Externally, they are used for their irritant effect on the skin. If used overzealously they will induce inflammation and blistering. Used judiciously, they increase blood flow into the area, helping to remove the build-up of waste products (cabbage poultices for mastitis or arthritic joints; mustard poultices for bronchitis). Taken internally, they can help to reduce thyroid function and are therefore potentially goitrogenic. Radish (*Raphanus sativus*), and mustard (*Sinapis alba et nigra*), *Armoracia rusticana* and *Tropaeolum majus* all contain significant amounts of glucosinolates. Internally they also are effective decongestants for sinus conditions and also simulate digestion, although large doses can cause vomiting. They also have some antibiotic and immunomodulant effects. Benzyl isothiocyanate, from the hydrolysis of glucosinolates, is found in *Tropaeolum majus* and is cytotoxic against human tumour cell lines.

Anthraquinones/Anthracene glycosides

Anthraquinones/Anthracene Glycosides are yellow-brown pigments with an aglycone of two or more phenols. It would appear that they pass through the stomach and small intestine unaltered, but they are converted into dianthrones in the caecum and colon by micro-organisms. They are then further converted into anthrone and anthraquinone which have laxative effects. This was formerly thought to be as a result of irritating the bowel mucosa, but it is now thought to be as a result of increased peristalsis and inhibition of water and electrolyte resorption by the mucosa. They normally take about 10 hours to produce a bowel movement and are therefore normally taken just before going to bed. They only work when bile is present. Examples are *Rhamnus catharticus, R. frangula, Rheum palmatum, Rumex crispus.* These species also contain tannins which moderate the laxative effect. *Aloe barbadensis* and *Senna sp.* are stronger in action. Herbs rich in these constituents are often combined with carminative herbs to reduce colicky or griping pains that can occur.

Hypericin in *Hypericum perforatum* is structurally an anthraquinone but does not breakdown in the bowel and has no laxative effect; *Hypericum* is known for its antidepressant and antiviral properties, for treating nerve pain and externally for healing damaged skin, in the form of an infused oil.

CHAPTER THREE

Plant families and their medicine

When learning about the herbs, it can be valuable to see which ones are grouped into the same family and notice that they often have similar characteristics—they may well look similar, smell similar, contain similar chemical constituents and have similar healing abilities or medicine. So, it is worthwhile to find out which herbs belong to the same family. Bear in mind that taxonomists sometimes change the names of the families and the individual plants and that nowadays taxonomical classification is done by DNA analysis whereas Linnaeus classified the plants by comparing flower structure amongst other things.

The list below is in no way complete as regards all the families that the plants belong to. It is also not complete as regards lists of plants in each family. However, it does allow the mentioning of many wonderful allies that did not find their way into the plant stories due to lack of space.

The exploration and investigation of the plant families is one that can really expand our awareness and happily gives us another excuse to explore with our green allies. Here are some examples of some therapeutically valuable families.

Apiaceae

The flowers are arranged in a flat umbel. The spokes of the umbel end in secondary umbels which bear a number of five-petalled flowers which are small and bisexual. The stems are hollow and ridged. The leaves are divided, compound, alternate and have no stipule. The ovaries are inferior, twinned and have two stigmas.

Anethum graveolens, Angelica archangelica et al, Anthricus cerefolium, Apium graveolens, Carum carvi, Coriandrum sativum, Cuminum cyminum, Daucus carota, Foeniculum vulgare, Hydrocotyle asiatica, Levisticum officinale, Pimpinella anisum, Petroselinum crispum.

Many have phytoestrogen effects, are stimulating nervines, carminatives and diuretics that help clear acid from the body via the urine.

Asteraceae/Compositae

Asteraceae/Compositae is the largest family. Their tiny flowers are closely packed into compound heads which are often mistaken for a single flower. The head is surrounded by sepal-like bracts. The florets are of two kinds—disc florets with the tube ending in five teeth, and ray florets around the edge of the head with a flat petal-like flap. Florets may be bisexual, unisexual or asexual. There is a collar of bracts beneath the flower head known as an involucre. The sepals are rings of hairs in many species known as a pappus. There are five fused petals, and five stamens forming a tube around the style. The ovary is inferior. Alternately arranged leaves (occasionally opposite); simple, compound and sometimes in a basal rosette. The fruits are achenes often with a persistent pappus to aid wind dispersal.

Bellis perennis, Calendula officinalis, Helichrysum italicum, Inula helenium, Lactuca virosa, Artemisia species, Achillea millefolium, Matricaria recutita, Silybum marianum, Solidago virgaurea, Tanacetum parthenium, Echinacea species, Taraxacum officinale, Arctium lappa, Tussilago farfara.

The therapeutics of this family are varied. For example, daisy, marigold, and immortelle are valuable skin remedies. Dandelion, yarrow, milk thistle, artemisias and elecampane are useful bitters.

Brassicaceae/Cruciferae

Brassicaceae/Cruciferae are annuals and perennials, which are not normally woody. The flowers have four petals arranged in a cross; usually six stamens in two whorls; four sepals. Flowers are usually stalked and in erect spikes or clusters. The ovary is made of two fused carpels. The seeds are in a beaked pod. The leaves are alternate with no stipules and are simple or pinnate. The aroma is pungent and sulphurous from the isothiocyanates. They taste bitter and pungent.

Cuckoo flower, mustard, bittercress, watercress, wild radish, *Capsella bursa-pastoris, Amoracia rusticana.*

This group are bitter and pungent and therefore are useful digestive tonics but can be emetic in excess. They are immune enhancing and probably benefit the gut flora. Some have a valuable warming action that reduces cold and damp in conditions like arthritis and bronchitis. Large amounts can suppress thyroid function.

Boraginaceae

Boraginaceae have a round stem and are rough and hairy. The flowers are usually blue, often pink, before opening. They have five joined petals and sepals, usually held in one-sided spikes that are tightly coiled initially. The sepals are long and hairy. The stamens are joined to the petal wall. The leaves are simple, undivided and alternate with no stipule. The ovaries are superior and have two carpels. The fruits are four nutlets.

Symphytum officinale, Pulmonaria officinalis, Borago officinalis.

These plants are mucilaginous. They can be valuable anti-inflammatories and help repair tissues. Some contain pyrrolizidine alkaloids (but not necessarily the ones that induce liver problems) but are safe when prepared by a method that uses heating and they also contain buffering substances that reduce the toxicity of these constituents.

Ericaceae

Evergreen shrubs and a few trees. Some such as bilberry are deciduous. The flowers have a distinct bell shape. The fruits are capsules or berries. All prefer acid soils except for *Arbutus*.

Cranberry, *Arctostaphylos uva-ursi, Calluna vulgaris, Vaccinium myrtillus* are all valuable urinary antiseptics.

Fabaceae/Leguminosae

Distinctive five-petalled flowers. The top petal is broad and erect, the two at the side are narrower wings, and the two lowest are joined as the keel which hides the stamens and styles. The flowers are mainly held in heads. The leaves are usually alternate, pinnate or trefoil and there maybe tendrils present. The roots have small nodules to house the nitrogen-fixing bacteria they are in symbiosis with. The fruit is a pod or legume. Legumes contain isoflavones and some alkaloids.

Trifolium pratense, Glycyrrhiza glabra, Medicago sativa, Galega officinalis, Trigonella foenum-graecum, Astragalus membranaceus, Cassia senna, alfalfa. Nutritive tonics and phytoestrogen-rich.

Lamiaceae/Labiatae

Lamiaceae/Labiatae are hairy or downy and may be annuals or perennials. They are often aromatic or pungent. The stems are square. The flowers have joined lipped petals and five sepal teeth. The flowers are usually held in whorls up the leafy stems. The leaves are opposite, toothed, usually stalked and undivided; they often have hairs or trivchoma. Fruits are clusters of four nutlets in a persistent calyx.

Ajuga reptans, Ballota nigra, Glechoma hederacea, Hyssopus officinalis, Lavandula vera/officinalis/angustifolia, Lamium album, Leonorus cardiaca, Lycopus europeus, Marrubium vulgare, Melissa officinalis, Mentha species, *Nepeta cataria, Origanum* species, *Prunella vulgaris, Rosmarinus officinalis, Salvia officinalis, Salvia sclarea, Scutellaria lateriflora, Stachys betonica, Thymus serphyllum et vulgaris.*

The members of this family all contain some level of volatiles oils which is what gives them their medicinal properties. Some are nervines, most are digestive tonics and carminatives, many are antimicrobial, and quite a few are expectorants and antispasmodics which support the respiratory system.

Onagraceae

Onagraceae are perennials, many with runners. The flowers are pink with four notched petals and undivided leaves. They frequently hybridise. The seeds have long plumes of silky hairs and are in long four-sided pods which split when ripe. Evening primrose, enchanter's nightshade, and rosebay willowherb all have nervine qualities.

Rosaceae

This family includes trees, shrubs and other forms. The flowers are very variable in size, but all have five petals and sepals, numerous yellow stamens and are bisexual. There is an epicalyx of sepal-like structures beneath the true sepals. The leaves are usually alternate, often compound with saw-toothed margins and stipules adhered to the leaf stalk. The carpels are free and numerous often in multiples of five. The receptacle is cup-shaped, with floral structures on the edge which may engulf the carpels. The fruits are usually compound, consisting of several to many achenes (dry) or drupes (fleshy).

Agrimonia eupatoria, Alchemilla vulgaris, Crataegus species, *Filipendula ulmaria, Fragaria vesca, Geum urbanum, Malus, Potentilla erecta, Prunus serotina, Rubus ideaus et fructicosus, Rosa* species.

They are tannin rich and the Prunus species contain cyanogenic glycosides.

CHAPTER FOUR

Wild gardening and a new paradigm of growing and harvesting

One role of humans in the ecosystem is in their service as gardeners.

We are all aware that some of the approaches we have taken to agriculture, horticulture, land use, forestry, food production and much more besides have not worked so well over the last while. However, there is an emergence of a desire to redress the balance to be more harmonious and responsible and to find solutions, to create a more constructive way of working with the land and other species with whom we share our places; solutions that make it a healthy place for all beings. At least, that is what a small but significant number of people who are reconnecting with our land are trying to do.

We are starting to look at focusing more locally, supplying our local markets, embracing concepts such as food sovereignty, medicine sovereignty and habitat restoration. It can seem overwhelming, especially if we search for blueprints in the wrong places. If we do that it can seem that there are no solutions to such big problems. However, if we do as Nature does and find similar places, use biomimicry, move our frontiers slowly and listen to the land and the ecosystems; if we remember that healthy ecosystem evolution occurs at the boundaries and that oxytocin really does boost repair, restoration and rejuvenation, and that we produce more oxytocin when we relax, then we relax into the work and go with the flow. Relaxation does not mean laziness; it means being calm and maintaining a smooth tone that allows the energy to build and flow.

In other parts of the world (Cuba, Bolivia, Bhutan, Portugal, Provence, Ecuador for example) they are rising to the challenges by seeing what can be restored from old wisdom and knowledge, what is valuable from the technologies and ideas of recent times and how to merge old and new in order to build a future that will work for us all. Most of the projects are small and community-based, arising from the community and its needs with a positive vision rather than one that seeks exponential growth, and that is driven by negativity and fear. We need to widen our approach from singly linear analytical approaches, to bring in more intelligences, to bring in creativity and use lateral thinking too. We need to listen and look to Nature for the solutions. Many of the so-called solutions being explored by the mainstream are being borrowed from sources that are not applicable. So, we need to find models and blueprints that are applicable to the land we live on; a small island with a diversity of native and naturalised species that can answer our challenges if we are creative in our thinking; we also have an excellent climate for welcoming some exotics that are helpful, and many of these have been grown here before.

Ireland used to have a rich medicinal and aromatic plant growing sector, growing herbs and medicinal plants and many other crops for export. In Ireland, we have one of the best stores of traditional plant knowledge in Europe thanks to the research carried out by the Folklore Commission in the 1930s, and much of this is documented in Gabrielle Hatfield's books. We also have many groups of people throughout the country who are starting to relearn old crafts and to re-invent them for the times we live in.

So, we can look at places where they have a culture of sustainable wild food and medicine foraging; countries that have incorporated the concepts of co-operatives in a wider perspective and adding value to ensure that all the individuals in the supply chain (including the plants) get a reasonable return for their work; look at countries like those in South America that have incorporated the concepts of rights for Nature and for the peasant population since we are all descendants of peasants and artisan).

We can start to explore potential ways of working with indigenous species sustainably as a way of creating environmental, ecological, social and economic capital; working with Nature rather than trying to dominate and impose; making cultivation and harvesting a work and way of life that enriches and enhances the ecosystem.

We can look at plant anthropology or ethnobotany with fresh eyes; rather than making these academic studies we can reconnect with ourselves, the land we live in and the other species that we share it with and explore from an ecocentric perspective rather than an anthropocentric one. And we can start to see the generosity of our habitat, being grateful for the gifts it shares rather than treating everything as resources to be consumed.

Food

Due to clever and rather cynical marketing, we have come to believe that functional foods, super greens and the like need to be exotic species and made in factories, nicely packaged into pills, capsules, bars and special products. Yet we have plenty of native species that are real superfoods and can be easily harvested in a sustainable fashion and used at home or to make artisan products in small to medium-sized enterprises. These include seaweeds, mushrooms, lichens, wild greens, berries, nuts, roots and much more. Actually, we have a great range of food plants growing all around us. Rather than growing modern cultivars, we can reclaim our heritage varieties, and our wild forage foods grow plentifully but are often treated as weeds rather than being used as beneficial foods full of micronutrients, antioxidants and all sorts of other things.

We can remember that animals fed on old pastures and mixed pasture are healthier and play an important part in mixed farming on small holdings and even on larger scale farms. Free range animals produce better meat, milk and eggs and are healthier and return their excrement to the land to feed that too. We can remember that old forest, mixed forest and natural forest grows more healthily (if more slowly) and contains all sorts of herbs, mushrooms and the like that can be wildcrafted sustainably. This in turn means that we have a healthier and more diverse insect, bird and mammal population. As well as remembering our own traditions we can look to places like Scandinavia, France and Italy and most of Eastern Europe and Russia where they have continued to use a wider diversity of plants.

It is quite amazing to realise that most herb teas sold here are imported from Eastern Europe, the Middle East or even New Zealand, including ones such as nettle and hawthorn that grow in such abundance. And many of our local plants such as blackberry are much fuller of antioxidants than green tea or other teas promoted as the ultimate source of such things; not to say that the exotics are not valuable, we have been trading herbs and spices with other regions for thousands of years but when we devalue our local food and plants at the expense of the exotics then we are out of balance. Before hops were introduced from Germany in the seventeenth century a much wider range of plants were used to make ale, gruit and beer; and many of these, such as spruce beer, were seen as medicinal foods or beverages. Hedgerow wines were produced from native berries and flowers and also were seen as tonics. We also have the potential to widen the range of culinary oils produced here. Rather than rapeseed oil (not a native and with undesirable environmental and health impacts), we could easily produce flax (there is now a company doing this), hemp, evening primrose, borage, blackcurrant seed, rose hip and many others.

There are endless possibilities of ways to broaden the diversity of what we grow and harvest, what we make from it and how to do this in harmony with the rest of the natural world rather than as an act of war against the soil and other beings. A side note is to realise that artificial fertilisers were only introduced after World War II when the munitions factories were threatened with closure since explosives were no longer needed in large quantity. Instead, they kept the factories open and rebranded the explosives as fertiliser. Similarly, most pesticides are biotoxins invented as biological warfare originally.

Medicine

Plants make medicines for humans and other animals, and to treat plants and the soil. Plants will make all of these healthier and can be used preventatively and curatively. We have so many valuable healing plants growing here that empower us to heal ourselves, the animals, our fields, gardens, plants and soil sustainably as we have been learning in our studies.

In the 1930s, one professor at University College Cork suggested that the Medicinal and Aromatic Plant growing sector be encouraged by the Department of Agriculture, alongside forestry and peatlands management. All three areas could do with revisiting. Coilte and the forestry division could be made significantly more sustainable, as could Bord ná Mona; and wildcrafting and growing medicinal and aromatic plant (MAP) crops would quickly help to revive rural social capital and provide small sustainable incomes for communities (they will never make fortunes, but then that is not what it is about; they could make an abundant supply of social capital though).

Textiles

Ireland used to have a booming flax and linen producing industry. Imagine all those fields of blue flowers again and flax ponds in each village. We could also revive harvesting nettles for the finest fibre, and there are some artisan companies now processing nettle for twine again. We could do this, rather than most of our clothes being made from imported textiles. We could grow hemp which provides fibre for textiles and for construction (the original design for the car used hemp fibre for the body), building materials, biofuels and the seeds for food; farmers used to be expected by law to grow some hemp before the petrochemical and nylon industry took off and it was made illegal to do so. There are other native and naturalised species that could be used for textiles and to provide alternative fibres for paper rather than using wood. It is also a good way to use the Japanese Knotweed and other species that have been maligned as invasive and destructive rather than being recognised as pioneers remediating the soil and providing great food and medicine.

Cosmetic and toiletries

These is another area where natural products can be used. There are now many artisan companies popping up that focus on using local and natural ingredients for skin care despite the fact the HPRA are bringing in all sorts of restrictions and rules about this. Then there are resins and glues and also pigments and dye plants to use for textiles and paints.

Habitat remediation

The area of habitat bioremediation is a huge one; planting reeds to clean up water polluted by effluent; using buckwheat, mushrooms and other species to clear heavy metals from polluted land and remediating clear cut bogs from around power stations by planting willows that can also be used as biofuel and will repair the land—using effective organism brews, repairing and re-inoculating with beneficial fungi and repairing the soil by stopping deep ploughing and using deep compost, huma- nure, and green manures for repair of our soils and stopping the use of agrichemicals, downscaling and increasing the human workforce on the land, reducing mechanisation. The possibilities are really endless and can inspire great creativity and positive solutions when one starts to explore. And remember it can be great fun!

Most of us are not working on that kind of scale and want to know how to work with the seeds and plants in a garden so we will look at this scale now. Anyone who has done horticultural or agriculture train- ing will normally learn a lot of techniques and information, and there are plenty of great sources of such information.

Once again, it is good to bring our feeling and listening, our sensing skills to this place, to make it into a conversation and become experien- tial and engaged on the journey with the plants.

We can work by feeling into the seeds, learning the song of the seeds, feeling what they need, feeding our information to them by sucking seeds, working with bare hands and feet and composting our waste to return to the soil. We can work with the plants when we are taking cut- tings by feeling into the plant, similarly with weeding and planting out. And when we are harvesting, we can ask permission, give gratitude and see what the plant and ecosystem wish to share with us, whilst making sure that as we harvest we are caretaking rather than pillaging.

Gardening as a metaphor

Growing plants, working with them holds some great metaphors for what we do in our lives and in healing ourselves:

Preparing and feeding the soil; Making sure that our own soils are healthy with enough structure, not too deeply dug, properly nourished and with a healthy microflora and proper composting of material that is used to feed the soil.

- Sowing seeds appropriate to the habitat.
- Saving and planting native seeds and those that suit our ecosystem.

- Freeing our garden of colonising weeds that might take over but recognising that some of those incomers may actually strengthen and improve the biodiversity of our ecosystem.
- Composting the weeds, leaves and other matter that is no longer needed.
- Making sure that our own nature gets what it needs to be a healthy ecosystem.
- Working with what we have to make our garden beautiful and dreaming and visioning making it more beautiful and healthy all the time.
- Making sure that we have sufficient biodiversity to create a healthy ecosystem.
- Allowing pollination to occur.
- Rotating crops and avoiding monoculture.
- Interplanting wild and cultivated species; making sure that all the levels of a forest garden are present.
- Giving time to take care of our garden properly, making sure that the unneeded, the bits that no longer serve are recycled and composted to add to the health of our garden or forest.
- Making sure that the plants are properly nourished and watered so that they do not get overrun by pests.
- Recognising which are pests and which are beneficial insects; their roles in pollination pest control and other aspects of ecosystem health.

It is good to explore these ideas as we look at growing herbs as our companions and allies in the work. There are also various methods of cultivation that include different philosophical approaches such as organic, permaculture, biodynamics, forest gardening, wild gardening, holistic gardening. They share some approaches in common and differ in some ways. They are all worth examining and exploring and seeing what resonates for one's own approach and the space that one is working with.

Growing from seed

There is a great pleasure to be had from watching a plant emerging from the seed and bringing it to maturity. By growing the plants yourself, nurturing them and getting to know their needs, you enter into a deeper relationship with them. You get to be able to recognise them from infancy to maturity. The same is true with wild plants; if you start to learn to identify them from the newly emerging seedling, through all their stages of development, you come to have a deeper understanding of your allies. For annual species, it is the most sensible way to raise plants—less cost and gives healthier plants. For many other species raising them yourself gives an intimate understanding of the plant and their nature. For non-native species, it is said that plants raised from seed are better adapted to the environment in which they find themselves, especially if they are the offspring of parents grown here. If the seeds you are planting are not poisonous and are uncoated (some companies coat seed with fungicides and other chemicals) then you may choose to suck them in your mouth before planting to exchange some of your information with them. Working with bare hands and walking barefoot on the soil you are working with enables you to send some of your physiological information into the soil (as well as enabling you to pick up the meanings from this amazing ecosystem). In this way, the plants and the soil receive another source of information about you and adapt their physiology into closer coherence with yours. The use of humanure further facilitates this process but may not be feasible unless you have a compost toilet and a sufficiently large area of land to enable you to use the compost on your growing areas.

Saving seed

Allow seed heads to dry out on blotting paper or newspaper to absorb any moisture, or by hanging them upside down in a paper bag. When heads are dry, shake out the seeds onto clean paper, remove any debris and store in a labelled envelope in a dry, cool place. Saving seeds can require regular trips out to check which seed heads are ready to harvest; it can be labour intensive. In the Irish climate, rain can impede the process; this is when seed may need to be harvested on damp days and gently dried on a tissue.

PART II

ENERGETICS, INTENTIONS AND MEDICINE

This part of the book focuses on intentions, the importance of evolving energetic understandings and their influences on the medicines we prepare from the plants.

CHAPTER FIVE

Evolving energetics

The energetics of any healing system describe how a particular culture believes or feels that healing energy flows; the different energy states of plants, people, the microcosm and macrocosm; how energy shifts in healing and in disease.

Biomedicine has a mechanomorphic system of energetics, the body as a machine. However, some practitioners and researchers in the current Western orthodox medical energetic model are slowing beginning to shift towards a more holistic and vitalistic view with new insights such as psychoneuroendocrinoimmunology, the re-emergence of the concept of the neuroendocrine system, the gut-brain microflora complex being elucidated and much more.

When people in the West want to explore energetics, they often tend to look towards models from other cultures such as Traditional Chinese Medicine (TCM) or Ayurveda, forgetting that we had a very rich system of energetics here in the form of Galenics for about 2000 years, alongside other traditional local ways of looking at healing. Still, as Caitlin Matthews says, it can be helpful to borrow embers from a neighbour when your own fire has died but only to help to get it going again; it is important to get one's own fire blazing again.

At the same time, what has tended to happen in systems such as Ayurveda and TCM is a degree of stagnation in old forms; energetics are about the flow of energy and therefore should evolve with changes in culture, and over time. So, at this point in time, it is valuable to examine widely what is described in other cultures, reach back to our own roots, compare what is similar and see what is different; even compare with the biomedical model and see how we get on with co-creating a new model.

As we start to examine how different cultures view energetics, we see that each system places different emphases; for example, in Ayurveda, energy is described as flowing through the chakras; whilst the TCM system talks about meridians. However, deeper examination shows that there are points analogous to the chakras in TCM and energy lines similar to meridians in Ayurveda.

As with so many areas, an understanding of current epistemologies is a useful starting place (borrowing embers from the neighbour), once one progresses the investigations and remembers to take a consilience view. As with everything else the most valuable approach as one looks at this area is to ask how it feels?

Relate the information back to your own body and being and see what resonates.

The qualities

Common to all systems of energetics is the concept of the four qualities:

- Heat and hot remedies possess the ability to purify, to refine, to eliminate alien substances.
- Cold, on the other hand, is the power to condense and bring things together. It is the cohesive power that can bind together things of opposite nature.
- Damp is a passive quality that allows flexibility and pliability and allows things to coerce. However, it is not easily contained due to its fluid nature. It will keep flowing until it dissipates unless there is a boundary.
- Dryness, on the other hand, sets boundaries and limits and therefore allows the creation of structure and function.

Each quality can be divided into four degrees, with four being the most intense and one being the least.

The five elements

For most energetics systems there are five elements that relate to the qualities:

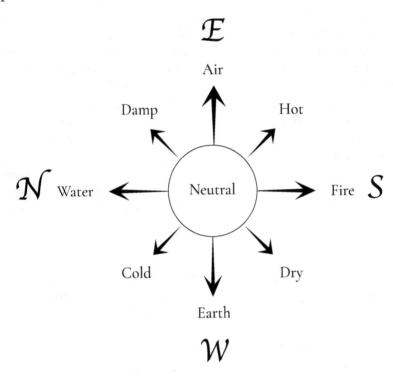

Galenics

Galenics was developed by Galen, AD 129–200, building on the Four Humours theory used in ancient Egypt and Greece.

The four Humours were first described by Hippocrates (460–370 BC):

- Blood
- Yellow bile
- Black bile (no physiological parallel)
- Phlegm

Galen developed this further into the Four Temperaments (from the Latin word temperare meaning to mix). Interestingly, people often find the concepts from this system easier to resonate with than the mechanomorphic lifeless model used nowadays. It retains the idea of vital force, vitality and the human as a living being.

Galen classified both people and herbs according to the Four Qualities, taken from the Four Elements, and related these and the Four Humours to the Four Temperaments.

The Four Temperaments are an integral part of Galenics, or the Western energetic system as used by herbalists like Culpeper. This system divides people into four archetypical types. A certain type might predominate at certain times of a person's life, and some people may swing between two types, being predominantly hot or cold or dry or damp. It could be argued that a balanced person expresses all four types in balance depending on age, circumstance, time of year and other internal and external factors. Alternatively, true balance may be perceived as the place of detached neutrality; probably, the truth is that energy and emotions flow therefore we do show signs of the various temperaments at different times, depending on the internal and external environment.

Sanguine

Sanguine's modern meaning is optimistic and confident, hearty. Literally bloody, the hot and moist blood humour is dominant.

Archetype: outgoing, lively, leadership qualities.

- Not always reliable.
- Prefers play to work, sociable and fun loving.
- Stable, cheerful, carefree, good-natured.
- Child-like, easily distracted.
- Quick minded, but sometimes shallow.
- Lives in the moment. Can be fickle.

Choleric

Choleric's modern meaning is irascible, liverish. Bilious, dominated by the hot, dry yellow bile.

Archetype: hot head.

- Extroverted and natural leader, independent and only yields to authority if it is respected. Intense, courageous, ambitious, optimistic, goal orientated.

- Eloquent and quick-witted, may be impatient and mocking and sometimes untruthful.
- Tends to be restless and excitable, even impulsive.
- May be touchy and aggressive.

Melancholic

Melancholic nowadays means depressed or pensive sadness, lung energy dominant. Cold and dry humour dominates—black bile which was thought to reside in the spleen.
Archetype: artistic temperament.

- Tends to introversion; very caring, understanding, sensitive and thoughtful.
- Tends to be quiet and responsible.
- The brooding artistic type—idealistic, deep thinking, takes life seriously.
- Can be anxious and moody.
- Reserved and unsociable.
- May be pessimistic, suspicious and solitary.
- Also, it can be rigid and obstinate in opinion.

Phlegmatic

Phlegmatic's modern meaning is stolid, calm, unexcitable and unemotional. A Splenetic type. Dominance of cold and moist phlegm.
Archetype: dull, lazy and sleepy.

- Persistent, reliable, reasonable and fair and with high principles.
- Tends to be introverted, stable, quiet, self-contained and placid.
- Modest and timid, prefers to stay with the familiar.
- Tends to be happy, simple.
- They are slow but shrewd.

There are several more layers that can be added to the elementary understanding. However, initially take time to observe people and see which temperament most closely describes them, or whether they move between one or more. Take time to taste, smell and feel into plants and foods and notice their qualities. Also take time to notice what activities and environments may help to nurture and build, or to deplete, the different temperaments, qualities and humours.

Now let's start to compare with other systems and the idea of flow. Energy flow is nicely illustrated by the chakra system, which many people have some familiarity with from yoga or meditation practice. It is important to understand that we are all unique and any intervention should be seeking to assist the individual to balance and harmonise rather than enforce an external manipulation.

Such descriptions also assume that the body is more than the physical entity that we are all aware of. Many people claim to or can see auras, and these can be photographed by the Kirlian method. The word aura comes from a Sanskrit root, meaning air, which in Latin means breeze. In ancient forms of medicine, it was believed that we are made up of four bodies or (seven).

The Spiritual body connects us to Unity. We are often unaware of this level of our existence.

The Mental body combines our ability to perceive concepts and our logical thought processes and memory.

The Astral body receives information about our environment and encompasses our mental body. It relates our personal experience to the Universe and contains the impressions of our life experience in thought forms. These are the colours that are seen within the aura. This body can be damaged, and areas of weakness may be seen as dents, or in extreme cases as holes.

As well as using colour, scent and sound, various forms of movement and meditation can be useful as means of strengthening our auric body.

Traditional chinese elements

In Chinese medicine, there is no element of ether, but they do use the term Chi which is more synonymous with vitality or life force, the vitality and capacity for activity. Each system and meridian has Chi, and one of the most important aspects is kidney Chi which is similar to the adrenal energy. It is made up of before-heaven Chi (what we get from our forebears, and what we are born with); and after-heaven Chi what we make during our lives influenced by nutrition, sleep exercise disease and so forth. It used to be taught that we could not repair or replenish our before-heaven or ancestral Chi, but this is not the case.

Signs of Chi deficiency are the same as the lack of vitality—fatigue, pale face, shallow breath or breathlessness, loose stools or a weak voice. We can consider how much energy we have overall (0 being totally flat, 10 being full Tigger bounce). We may notice that there are particular times of day when we feel more tired, and this can give a clue to which meridians and elements need healing and restoring. We can notice how much energy we have when we wake in the morning and whether we feel we have the energy to do what we need and wish to during the day.

Other disharmonies of chi include rebellious chi and chi stagnation. Rebellious chi includes sneezes, coughing, prolapse, reflux, vomiting and hiccups and this is similar to vapours rising in the physiomedical tradition.

When Chi becomes obstructed or stagnant, it can cause illness or discomfort in a particular area or as a more general condition in the body from repressed emotions. These can manifest as feelings of fullness, discomfort, swellings, pain, a sense of blockage in the throat or irritability, which come and go.

Yin and Yang

Yin and Yang are used to describe how seemingly opposing forces are interconnected and interdependent in the natural world, giving rise to each other in turn. Many natural dualities, e.g. dark and light, female and male, low and high are thought of as Yin and Yang. However, remember that in the Yin and Yang symbol there is a small dot of Yang in Yin and of Yin in Yang and the symbol shows how each flows into the other, creates the other; it is a spiralling cycle.

- Yin and Yang can manifest as deficient or excessive.
- Excess yang is indicated by restlessness, insomnia, fidgeting, tremors.
- Excess yin is indicated by quiet behaviour, desire to be immobile or sleepiness.

Traditional Chinese Medicine divides energy into five elements also referred to as transitions or the five transformations. It is helpful to look at them as phases that move rather than fixed definitions; they are Earth, Water, Metal, Fire and Wood. In this system, description of energy flow is inspired by natural cycles.

The cycle of creation

Wood creates Fire by providing fuel; Fire feeds Earth by providing ash; Earth creates Metal by providing ore; Metal creates Water by being smelted into the liquid state; Water feeds Wood

The cycle of control

Wood controls Earth (trees secure the soil); Earth controls Water through providing the foundation for streams and rivers; Water controls Fire through dampening flames; Fire controls Metal by smelting ore: Metal controls Wood through the ability to cut down trees.

Wood

Wood is described as rising Yang; spring; morning; liver and gall bladder; spirit, ethereal soul (Hun); anger; highest expression is compassion. Sour herbs feed wood.

The wood element is like a willow tree, flexible, resilient and powerful. It helps to think of the sap rising in the spring, that burst of sudden growth, the power contained in the bud of a plant. The liver governs the connective tissue of the body and allows for flexibility giving grace to movement. It is also the driving force of action, to go forward in life. It has a sense of purpose, of vision or plans. It allows us to get what we want from life; if this does not happen, it leads to frustration and anger. It is a very powerful force to be blocked; if this happens stagnation results.

This burst of spring growth arises from the energy stored over winter; however, this cannot be maintained. Wood is expressed by creativity and direction in life. If plans are thwarted, frustration and anger may arise. Anger gives us the force and power to break through blockages, giving us the determination to achieve our goals. Anger turned inwards may affect the joints or turn to destructive behaviour. The liver governs the quality of the blood, when lying down the blood is stored in the liver. It controls rhythm in the body, especially the menstrual cycle.

You can nourish your liver by stretching which eases out stagnation, improves flexibility and benefits the joints. Sideways stretches benefit the liver especially and help to reposition the organs.

The sour flavour stimulates contraction and absorption. It has a gathering or astringent action. It helps to treat leaking or sagging conditions involving loss of body fluids such as sweating, diarrhoea or haemorrhage. It counteracts the effect of fatty foods, prevents stagnation and benefits digestive absorption. It alkalises the body and stimulates secretions from the gall bladder and pancreas. Foods and herbs that have the sour flavour are generally cleansing and detoxifying. Lemon, lime, purslane, hibiscus, rosehip, sumac, vinegar and tamarind are sour. Dark green foods such as spinach and kale help to nourish the liver, whilst cleansing the system at the same time.

Fire

Fire is radiant Yang, summer, midday, heart, pericardium, small intestines and triple heater; spirit-mind (shen); joy, highest expression—love. Bitter herbs feed fire.

The fire element resides in the heart and is said to be the seat of consciousness or mind. Strong fire energy can be seen in the eyes, the complexion and the gesture of the hands. It has a radiant quality to it, with healthy emotions and is nourished by connection to other people.

The heart gives quality to the voice. Speech impediments are said to be connected to the heart; especially stammering and stuttering. Weak heart energy may cause a feeling of disconnectedness, leading to chest pain, insomnia, agitation, confusion or over-excitement.

You can nourish your heart and improve your fire energy by paying attention to your voice, by singing, chanting, humming, praying or using mantra meditations. Also pay attention to your voice, enjoying its quality, taking care with the words you choose and laughing.

The bitter flavour is draining and drying. It travels downwards in the body, improving appetite, stimulating digestion, drawing out dampness and heat. In excess, it can deplete Qi and moisture. Fenugreek, parsley, coffee, oregano orange peel, cocoa, artemisias, dandelion root, chicory, elecampane, vervain, ground ivy and many other herbs have bitter elements to them. Dandelion root stimulates the heart. Bitter elixirs such as aperitifs taken before a meal stimulate the digestive system to nourish the heart.

Earth

Earth descending Yin; late summer/Indian summer; afternoon; stomach and spleen/pancreas; spirit—intellect (Yi); emotion—reflection; highest expression—empathy. Sweet herbs feed Earth.

The earth element resides in the spleen (spleen-pancreas). It allows us to take in nourishment from the world, transforming food into usable substances for the body. A strong spleen ensures that a person is well nourished. Conversely, a weak spleen may mean that a person can consume a healthy meal and not have the capacity to transform it into nourishment. The spleen gives the body the capacity to hold up the tissues; if it is weak, it can lead to sagging such as a flabby belly or prolapse (typically varicose veins).

It also transforms and processes information and knowledge. Earth is the element of thought and gives us the ability to concentrate. Similarly, over-thinking or worry is a pathological condition of the earth element. The archetype of the mother is related to spleen energy, whereby a child's needs are provided by mother. Often food can distract people from their true emotional needs.

The sweet flavour is the most common of all foods; it harmonises other flavours and is deeply nourishing and moistening. It may be divided into full or empty sweetness. Full includes most meat, legumes, nuts, dairy and starchy vegetables: it is considered strengthening. Empty-sweet is contained in most fruit and sweeteners and is considered cooling and cleansing. The sweet flavour is often eaten to excess causing dampness. If food is chewed thoroughly, it will increase the sweet flavour; this is true for whole foods. Thoroughly chewing your food is one of the easiest ways to support your spleen function. Liquorice is a sweet flavoured, moistening herb that tonifies digestion and promotes absorption. Others include *Codonopsis* and *Asparagus racemosus*; dandelion and burdock roots also have some sweetness.

Metal

Metal gathering Yin; autumn; evening; lung and large intestine; spirit—bodily soul (P'o); grief; highest expression—reverence. Pungent herbs feed metal.

Metal makes a boundary or a border, physically through the skin and lungs. Having this boundary or surface allows for full interaction with the environment. Having a clearly defined boundary gives a greater sense of self and improves our relationship with others, enabling us to say yes to what we want and no to what we don't want. It is traditionally related to the father archetype, which defines self-worth and our place in the world. Self-esteem on the positive side, or the lack of it, which leads to sadness and depression.

The action of the breath is our most basic and immediate interaction with the world. This also allows the process of taking in and letting go. The organs of the metal element are the lungs and large intestine; thus, at the physical level, metal is expressed by the lungs, skin and colon. The lungs here refer to all of the respiratory system including the nose and sinuses. The skin also breathes and exchanges substances with the world. The large intestine or colon is a primary releasing organ.

Strong lungs give a strong physical vitality, healthy breathing and a clear, powerful voice. If the lungs are weak, there will be low vitality and a weak immune system. There may be shallow breathing, a weak voice. Emotionally there may be low self-esteem, sadness or an inability to claim a rightful place in the world.

The pungent flavour disperses and promotes circulation. It stimulates digestion and helps to break down mucus. Herbs include cayenne, chilli, clove, cumin, coriander, horseradish, rocket, onion and mustard.

The lungs or metal element are nourished through breathing exercises and meditation. Paying attention to the quality of the breath without trying to change it throughout the day, helps to focus on the metal element, doing specific meditations to increase our awareness and capacity to breath, engaging different parts of our lungs can increase our vitality.

Water

Water condensed Yin; winter; kidney and bladder; spirit will (zhi); fear; highest expression—wisdom. Salty herbs feed water

Water is the start of life and the foundation for our bodies. In TCM, the kidney is at the root of all functioning of the body, the source of Fire and Water. The water element expresses the most basic activity of survival: reproduction, growth and fight-or-flight response (fear or courage). It is the closest connection to our ancestors from whom we inherit our constitutions. Associated with the bones, teeth, brain, lower back and knees. The kidneys govern the reproductive organs, and govern the drainage and balancing of the fluids in the body.

Strong kidney energy is indicated by a strong reserve of life force, we may tire but the batteries don't run out. After sufficient rest, our energy is renewed. Reactions should be quick, the mind alive, alert and curious like a child, the pelvic area should be warm and loose and the spine strong and supple. Imbalances in the water element can lead to fear, reproductive disturbances, urinary system problems, or problems with the back, knees, ears, teeth or hair. Kidney imbalances are often indicated by dark blue/black circles under the eyes or a feeling of lack of support such as low backache.

The salty flavour moves inwards and downwards drawing the action of herbs towards the centre of the body. It softens, moistens and detoxifies counteracting the hardening of muscles and glands. It regulates moisture balance in the body by draining excess moisture as well as remoistening the body in conditions of dehydration. It stimulates digestive function and improves concentration. An excess of salt can congeal the blood and stress the heart. Seaweeds, nettle, parsley helps to nourish the kidneys, as does wearing a kidney scarf around the lower back area. Rubbing the kidney area to generate warmth then holding your hands over that area.

The seven directions and the celtic medicine wheel

The concept of the medicine wheel and the wheel of the year is existent in most indigenous medicine systems although each has slightly different correspondences. We will focus on the local one. Some people assign particular animals and plants and mythic persons to the directions although there is a large degree of local variation and to some extent this is a personal thing.

East

The rising sun or morning, wisdom, air, new beginnings and the child and possibilities, spring.

South

The midday sun, knowledge, fire, action, youth, summer.

West

The setting sun or evening, understanding, earth, manifestation, dreaming, incubating and being, adult, autumn.

North

The broad night, sky night, water, reflection and surrender, elder, winter.

The centre

The land of spirit, ether, vitality, being present in the here and now.

Above

The sun, the moon, the stars and the planets.

Below

The Earth and all her creatures, both seen and unseen.

Within this wheel, we see the presence of the wheel of the year, the cycles of the day and the cycles of life. You may notice some similarities, and also differences, to the elements in the Chinese cycles. This is because both are based on observances of the cycles of Nature in a temperate region.

Seasons and cycles

At each time of the year, the plant world provides what is needed. Tomatoes protect against sun damage. Many evergreens help with lung energy—ivy, cedar, pine, laurel, cypress, holly. Nettles and dandelions leaves, dock leaves work as a spring tonic. Primrose for spring coughs, elderberries for building the immune system for winter, elderflower for hay fever and so forth. Root vegetables contain inulin for immunity in winter. But we need to remember that this provision is not just for the humans. The plants are working on each other, the soil, the air, the water, the insects, animals and the invisibles too; so, we thank Nature and the plants for their generosity and ask permission, ask whether they are providing for us or for others.

We are part of the web—as the seasons change so do we with them, so does the rest of Nature, so does the Earth. And this makes sense of eating local food that is in season, or that has been preserved from our locality. Our physiology changes—making sense of the TCM cycle of the year. So, in the winter months, we need to deal with our deepest fears as we are surrounded by the dark. We step into the dark places and bring forth the shadows so that they can be brought into the light. This results in wisdom. As we move into the spring, we feel the sap rising in the wood, and we can become angry as the energy rises—anger gives us the energy to change things, to detoxify and deal with all those emotions and ideas that have become trapped in our liver. Anger gives us the energy to shift all the confusion in the gall bladder so that our ideas can flow, and we can plan clearly. And then we move into compassion for ourselves and the world around us. As the heat of summer arrives, we feel the joy that comes with this; we can fall in love with the world. As the Indian summer arrives, we start to reflect on the world and ourselves; as we reflect, we can become empathic. Then we move into the autumn, to metal and the time of grieving, when we grieve well we can move into reverence.

By eating in tune with the cycle, we help to attune ourselves to the shifts and changes that naturally occur in the year; we can make the web healthier. By working with the rhythms of the day we also make our rhythms healthier, and by working with the rhythm of our life cycles too.

There are many other systems of energetics to explore in this reweaving, evolution, revolution. There are many ways to ascertain, diagnose or recognise the energetic balance within a person, plant or place.

The three cauldrons

In pre-Christian Celtic energetics, there was also the oral tradition of the Three Cauldrons. This was first recorded in written form by an Irish fili or sacred poet in the seventh century in *The Cauldron of Poesy*. Filidh were often associated with monasteries, until at least the seventeenth century, when the English began earnest attempts to destroy Irish Catholicism. Caitlin Matthew's translation of this manuscript and analysis thereof in the *Encyclopaedia of Celtic Wisdom* is perhaps the most accessible.

Put simply:

The Lower Cauldron (Coire Goirath) is known as the cauldron of warmth or incubation and is centred in our pelvis like the lower burner or Hara of Eastern Medicine philosophy. We are born with this cauldron upright, a bowl of vitality which gives us our physical, health, mobility and life force.

The Lower Cauldron needs to be full, relaxed and nourished in order for us to survive and thrive both as an individual and then as a species. When it is full, it provides heat and energy for our whole being and allows the Middle Cauldron to fill.

The Middle Cauldron or Coire Ernmae is known as the cauldron of vocation and motion. It is positioned in the centre of the chest in the heart region. All our life experiences of joy and sorrow cause it to turn and fill so that we can walk our vocational path and in time fill our Upper Cauldron.

The Middle Cauldron is about our connection to our community, our emotional wellbeing and our heart star healing capacity; knowing our life path and following it, centred in our community.

We produce a particular form of energy here which is part of our ecological function; it is the energy of compassion and caring and bonding in the community. We also give, receive and process a lot of our emotional intelligence and information in this cauldron. This may well be the cauldron that both produces and receives awen.

The Upper Cauldron or Coire Sois is the cauldron of wisdom, knowledge or inspiration and is located in the centre of the head around the third eye. For many people, this cauldron is upside down unless they have done the emotional work of filling the second cauldron. Once this is done, we can turn this cauldron upright and start to fill it.

This our cauldron of connection to spirit and our psyche. Although our mental and spiritual faculties are spread through our being, as are our physical and emotional, it is generally agreed that in order to be healthy, well-grounded and embodied we first fill our Lower Cauldron, then our Middle and finally our Upper one.

CHAPTER SIX

Intentions in medicine making; the wild kitchen and pharmacy

T he way in which a medicine is prepared from a plant will have an effect on the way it expresses itself (in part due to the actual constituents, the matter that is extracted and also due to the interactions that occur during the preparation process). The overall meaning and medicine of the plant, for example, *Avena* (oats), will be there but maybe certain aspects of its personality will come through more strongly, depending on the way it is prepared, who is giving the medicine and who is receiving it.

It also depends on the part of the plant that is used, where it grew, with what other plants it shares in community (plants such as opium poppy secrete their alkaloids into the soil and have a relaxing effect on the plants in their community, for example); how it was harvested (it is generally considered that lavender essential oil prepared from flowers handcut in the traditional manner is vastly superior to the oil prepared from whole plants grubbed up by machines). We explored this a little more when we talked about cultivation, harvesting and processing but suffice to say that the more we ask permission, set clear intentions from a place of integrity, and communicate with the plant as to what we intend to use the medicine for, whether it is to use for yourself or for use with a wider community, the better the medicine given by the plant. Each plant is an individual of its species that expresses that species in its own unique way, in the same way that each human expresses *Homo sapiens sapiens* in their own way—physically, emotionally, spiritually. Physiological shifts that manifest with healing are the physical expression of the shifts that are happening on a spiritual level.

We are following a green thread

We are blessed with a plethora of books full of information about the active constituents in plants, clinical and research evidence, traditional uses and much more. All that information is very valuable, but we need to take the information and turn it into knowledge and then let that knowledge mature into wisdom.

I have been working with the plants for many years and deepening a relationship with them by sitting with them, engaging sensory acuity by looking, tasting, smelling, touching and by listening to them. The plants are the real teachers in this work and also my students pushing me to dig deeper.

One of my students made an extremely important point: the plant works to heal not by treating a particular symptom, or symptom set, but by feeding in meanings that align the person to the essential character of the plant. She made this point when we were discussing wood betony in class, and I mentioned how I had had a discussion about its therapeutic application with a colleague, and she said she used it for the exact opposite to what I used it for. When she said that I looked at the plant again and saw how it has really strongly grasping roots, a rosette of beautifully scalloped leaves hugging the ground and then throws up a slender stem (sort of wiggly, like the vagus nerve), at the end of which appears a spike of deep pink flowers. Wood betony anchors us down to the earth, balances the vagal tone and the heart energy, it is traditionally described as driving away fear—what better way to do this than to be grounded and connected to the heart? But that is just an energetic explanation of all the other things that it does and the specific therapeutic actions it possesses, and this is a very important part of understanding the meaning of wood betony.

The plant aligns the person with its medicine, it's personality; we need to take this to deeper levels of understanding; a more profound realisation of the fact that herbs bring particular tissues, systems, personality aspects into alignment, into health, that they bring new meanings into us to help us become more fully whom we were born to be.

The profound wound of the Western world, the removal of the spirit and soul from the material world, the view of the Universe (and therefore plants and people) as a machine has to some extent snuck into our supposedly vitalistic and holistic practice. Furthermore, the militaristic attitudes of the dominator model that permeates the West also seems to have filtered in. Most of us would agree with the principle of using herbs to strengthen our terrain, or soil, to build vitality; most of us agree that we do not want just to treat symptoms or kill off the invaders; most of us would agree that we would like to reweave energetics back into herbal medicine and be part of co-creating and co-evolving this process with the plants who offer their medicine. Each plant has its core medicine; it's multidimensional personality. For those of us who sit with plants in conversation, we start to meet the soul, the spirit of the plant, to get to know them as allies and friends who help us to heal; we listen to them and are also conveyors of their medicine to the people who need them, we are in service to their medicine. Although research into herbs is valuable and can help elucidate the way a plant works, we need to remember that science is a tool, not a god, not a master, but a servant, as we all are. Science is not purely objective; it is affected by outcome expectations. Science is one way of describing a plant's medicine. It does not validate the plant or make it valuable, they are already; science and research just help to confirm the intrinsic value of the medicine these sentient beings offer to us.

Unfortunately, what has happened with a lot of research is that a particular plant becomes known as the one for treating colds and flus (*Echinacea*, elderberry), treating migraine (feverfew), repairing the liver (*Carduus*). All the other aspects of the work they do are often lost; we tend to get stuck in a superficial categorisation of their personality, their medicine. Most people I know do not enjoy being discounted and put in a box like that. So often herbal training involves getting a superficial acquaintance with 200–300 allies, rather than a profound relationship with 20–30. How many of us are capable of really knowing 200 people? It is better to know 40 things about 1 plant than to know 1 thing about 40 plants. It would appear that at the moment many plants are beginning to speak up for themselves and call our attention to the fact that we have been completely ignoring them as weeds, or as rather insignificant local, outdated beings that have been superseded by the exotic exciting new favourites, often from overseas, often packaged as products.

The point is that plants have never just worked on a physical level. Even when they are prescribed purely for physical symptoms they work physically, emotionally, mentally, spiritually; they must do because they are conscious, sentient, multidimensional complex beings just like us. I remember someone once saying to me that herbs are used for physical ailments but that one needs a vibrational preparation such as a flower essence or homoeopathic remedy to shift emotional and spiritual issues. From what the plants around me are saying that is just not true. We need to breathe the soul back into our medicine. The plants do this anyway, but if we work with this consciously it means that we can match up plants and people far more elegantly, and it means that our medicine becomes soul medicine; like the way food is described as soul food in places like New Orleans and the Caribbean—nourishing on all levels, filled with love. The plants are doing the work on this level anyway, they are sentient and conscious and know this; if we step into work with them in this way, how much more healing and sacred medicine flows to heal the World soul, our cultural soul, to bring about a more sacred alignment between our species and the rest of the beings in our world and on the Earth.

For example, so often we prescribe *Echinacea* for colds and flus (because it kills viruses). A rather militaristic view. *Echinacea* has been shown to kill off some viruses and some bacteria. However, if we want to take a more community-based, sustainable view of how herbs work their medicine, we need to dig a little deeper, see what else this amazing plant does? It does not just kill off viruses, and bacteria, it helps to prevent them from breaking through our cell walls to replicate by inhibiting an enzyme called hyaluronidase. This means it is also good for preventing the body from breaking down its own connective tissue in autoimmune disease (conditions where our immune system fails to recognise our own tissue as self). In general, it helps with tissue repair, especially epithelial tissue and with cartilage because it prevents hyaluronidase from breaking down the tissues. It is a wonderful lymphatic herb, helping to get rid of waste in the body. As a root full of polysaccharides, it is also likely to be a nourishing tonic. Echinacea reduces inflammation (a core issue with most chronic disease), increases saliva production, stimulates healthy antibody production and both stimulates and modulates the immune system. It is also excellent for nervous fatigue.

Added into the therapeutic process are other factors: the intentions of those preparing and dispensing the medicine, and the medicine that they put into the process will affect the outcome. The medicine of the person ingesting the preparation; in any healing process, there is an interaction between the person seeking healing, the person holding the healing space and the medicine itself.

The other factor that needs to be considered is what other plants are taken at the same time; there is the practical consideration of which constituents may interact with each other, but also there is the consideration of what therapeutic affect is being looked for on all levels. There is no generalised right or wrong approach as to whether to take plant medicines as simples or in complex formulae, once one considers the needs for a particular person at a particular place and time. What we need to consider is that each plant is bringing information and meanings into the body; in order to effect a true healing shift, those meanings need to be embedded so that the entrainment that occurs can be habituated, making the shift a lasting one. This means that sometimes a complex blend of herbs may be what is needed, but at other times a single herb is what is required. The number of doses and the size of the dose to allow entrainment will vary from person to person and will also vary for an individual at different times and in different circumstances. What this means is that we need to listen carefully to the plants and to the person seeking medicine, we need to be present and not make assumptions.

We are all aware of the fact that we bring forward different aspects of our personality when interacting with different people or groups of people and in different scenarios. Plants do the same thing; so, although there may be broad similarities in the therapeutic effects of lavender from individual plants of the species, *Lavandula officinalis* works on most humans, there will also be variations, nuances. In the same way that not all people get on together (however wonderful we are, our medicine does not always blend well with that of equally amazing people), part of the skill of working with the plants is to listen to them with regard to the specific person who is seeking medicine, to the time and the situation you are working with—there are no absolutes. We deepen our relationship and knowing of the plants, incorporating information such as their constituents, their properties, their general uses, and we also sit with them to deepen our relationship with them, and we continue to do this as we do with dear friends, with people in our community. We deepen our relationship with them so that when we are asked to we can match up that sacred knowledge with what we read from the person asking for assistance; we listen to the person's story clearly and we never make assumptions.

To put it another way: the plants are our allies, particular plants become our special allies, and then there are those that we work with less often, our acquaintances. This is similar to the way we have close friends amongst our own species, but also a wider circle of acquaintance with whom we interact from time to time; and there are those that we know we do not work well with and those with whom we have a more challenging relationship. So, the plants are our allies and our teachers. We need to get to know them on every level and to ask them how we can work with them.

For certain plants you may work with them in many forms, others you may find you only work with one particular form. For example, you may find that you use Lavender only as an essential oil, whilst you use rose as an aromatic water, and a tincture, and an essential oil, and a fixed oil and a food-medicine. We need to remember that we bring our own medicine and offer it alongside the medicine of the plant and that it is part of our work to continue to rigorously examine ourselves and to bring our medicine into more coherence, into a more sacred alignment with the medicine of the *Anima Mundi*. We reach beneath the surface to find meanings ever deeper; the meanings of ourselves and of the plants.

How sustainable is our medicine?

If we are truly on the path of plant medicine, then we need to let go of our anthropocentric arrogance and remember that the healing is for the planet and our harvesting and preparation of the herbs must be both consensual and sustainable, promoting biodiversity and planetary health as well as our own.

One day, we were discussing what herbs to use for treating tooth abscesses in class. One of the students suggested *Hydrastis*, and I said that I did not tend to use *Hydrastis* and preferred to use *Berberis vulgaris*. Another of the students asked why I did not like *Hydrastis*. It is not that I do not like *Hydrastis*; it is a beautiful plant and a beautiful being. I love it and respect it and never work with it in herbal prescriptions. Why? Because it has been pillaged from its natural habitat to a horrifying extent, in the same way that virtually no *Echinacea* of the 20 odd species remain in the prairies of the US (I do use *Echinacea* but only from cultivated sources and only when I cannot find a substitute).

In contrast, *Berberis vulgaris* has a far wider range, is native to Europe and reasonably widely cultivated as a hedging plant and is therefore not under pressure or endangered. As a European native the ecosystem that it has evolved in is far closer to that of our patients in Europe, it has co-evolved in a similar habitat and therefore may well provide medicine that is more in line with our own physiology (if you live in a place where it does not grow there are likely to be plants that grow where you are that are high in berberine and the other constituents that make this plant such good medicine such as *Berberis aquifolium, Coptis chinensis, Corydalis sp., Tinospora cordifolia*).

Hydrastis has been brought into cultivation in some areas of the US, Ireland, Scotland and other places, and there is a place for using such sources, without a doubt. However, a plant in its natural habitat does not just provide medicines for humans, it plays an intrinsic role in its community, providing for birds, animals, insects, other plants, the soil and its microflora—it is in an intimate relationship with many other beings. So, when we plunder a community in this way, we really are acting out the worst of crimes. I do not see how we can stand over such behaviour if we are truly wishing to be herbalists, caring about sustainable, holistic medicine. I feel that we need to ask forgiveness for those acts; even if we did not carry them out, we need to recognise the responsibility our species carries as a whole for such egocentric, anthropocentric, immature vandalism. People argue that *Hydrastis* has now been brought into cultivation and therefore the responsible consumer can use these sources; this is true.

However, there is one part of me that feels very strongly that surely if such damage has been done and we learn how to cultivate these plants we should first seek to remediate what has been done; repopulate the areas that have had one of their kin exterminated, restore the aftermath of our genocide; I am purposefully using quite emotive terms and language in these musings since I feel we really need to be shaken out of our complacency about some of the wounds we have perpetrated, and that we need to be clear about exactly what our anthropocentric hubris has done to the rest of Nature. Gary Snyder said, 'Nature is not a place to visit, it is home'. So how would we feel about families, communities, homes where this kind of behaviour to kith and kin was seen as acceptable, as normal? Anyone who has been reared in a home or community where such abusive behaviour was seen as just grand, fine, par for the course knows that it is not.

I have heard practitioners say that since they have been taught how to use these plants, they have the right to continue dispensing them—that sounds dubious, extremely immature and unconscious; the attitude of the spoiled child.

I have heard practitioners argue that each plant has its own special healing niche and therefore they should continue to be able to use them. It is true that each plant has its own unique character, but surely it is therefore most important for it to be present in its native community where it provides healing for other members of its own species, other plants, the soil, the insects, the animals, where it sings its own part in the choir, plays its own part in the orchestra of that natural harmony?

Human beings have a particular ability to be creative in their choices; if a particular plant has been ravaged then surely we have the intelligence and ingenuity to substitute other plants, to go back to the creative drawing board and make another match for the person stepping forward to ask for healing from the plants? Surely that is part of the essence of true herbalism, to reach towards a healing that cures those wounds to the sacred so that the human species no longer experiences separation from the whole, no longer feels separate from Nature but rather steps back into its ecological function within Nature?

We can also feel into what the initial plant is telling us about the person and is part of that person's story similar to the story of *Hydrastis* as regards the wounding it has experienced—and so what other herbs are good for that particular kind of wounding. Or where does *Hydrastis* naturally grow, what is its song in regard to being at home in the shade of the trees in deciduous forest, truly at home in a mature ecosystem where infants (saplings), mature adults and elders are not separated out but rather live in a whole community of all ages and of different species?

It seems to me that true herbal medicine does not just concentrate on the wounds of the human species but reaches beyond this to see the externalised wounds that we have created. From that place, we can do our inner work, heal the microcosm and then, in health, reach out to heal the macrocosm.

A truly skilled herbalist can learn to listen to the story of a person, hear the first plant that steps forward, and then hear that plant's story; listen to whether that plant's history further illuminates the patient's story: does the call to use *Hydrastis* mean that the person has experienced similar in their life or is it the only herb that will help them?

The sorrow, grief, and rage you feel is a measure of your humanity and your evolutionary maturity. As your heart breaks open, there will be room for the world to heal.
Joanna Macy: Greening of the Self

Simple, effective, affordable and sustainable methods of making herbal medicines

We live in interesting times. The rise of austerity is pressing on many people, and they need to be empowered to look after the health of themselves and their communities. The health of our ecosystems is being decimated by capitalism too. We need solutions, and we need them fast and affordably—plant medicine is a wonderful solution. We have a vision of community clinics where people gather together in meitheal style to prepare and share medicines made from locally tended plants, to build community, remediate our landscapes and ecosystems and build healthy solutions, some awen and oxytocin. Silvia Frederici talks about the value of restoring the commons in her book *Re-Enchanting the World* and this is something I feel passionate about. Therefore, the methods below are described simply enough to teach anyone and are mainly made from extremely affordable and local ingredients which can be made at home (so no glycerine). This is what we base most of our practice on (hence our nickname of the radical pesto makers—one of the best ways of getting large quantities of herbs into a person), although we do use some essential oils and some exotic herbs.

Food-medicine

One of the simplest and oldest ways of using herbs is to eat them as food. Hippocrates said: let your food be your medicine and your medicine be your food; well, we can really do this with herbs. Dieting on herbs is a most excellent form of preventative medicine, a way of connecting properly with our environment, making ourselves more aligned with Nature, part of Nature. Herbs are full of all sorts of nutrients which are antioxidant, anti-inflammatory, immune system and tissue building, cleansing and a tonic to the blood, clearing for the liver and much more besides. Studies are emerging showing that including forage foods and good quantities of herbs and spices in the diet are preventative and curative for most of the ills of Western culture such as diabetes, high blood pressure, high cholesterol, chronic inflammatory disease in general.

Kids love the frisson of preparing food from 'weeds' and wild plants. Many of our most valuable native and naturalised plants can be included in the diet easily and are much easier to grow than the cultivars that we tend to eat; they are fresher, in season, totally local and are really flavoursome.

Teas, tisanes or infusions

Teas, tisanes or infusions are probably the next oldest way of using herbs, and definitely one of the easiest ways of using them. They are generally prepared from leaves, flowers, aerial parts and some seeds, either fresh or dried; they can also be prepared from powders of harder plant parts such as roots, barks and seeds. Teas will mainly extract the water-soluble components of the plant. If you are using an aromatic plant (one containing essential oil) use a teapot, or place a saucer over the cup whilst infusing. Always use freshly boiled water. Some plants are used as a substitute for tea, and up to 5 cups can be safely consumed in a day. However, I would recommend that if being used in this way a maximum number per day would be 3–4 for any single herb, and to use a variety of herbs from day to day or during the day, rather than just one (unless you are dieting with a particular plant to get to know it better). Some herbs are much stronger in their action, not really suited for food use, and should be taken less often in the day.

The standard way to prepare a tea is to use 1 tsp dried herb or 2 tsp fresh herb (or a mixture of herbs) for 1 cup; pour on boiling water and allow the herbs to infuse for 5–10 minutes. If you are preparing a pot, use 20 g dried herb or 30 g fresh herb to 500 ml water. Infusions can be stored in a covered container in the fridge for up to 24 hours. They may also be made in a thermos flask and stored in this for 24 hours.

Do not add milk as this may bind some of the active constituents. Try to take without sweetening since the taste of the herbs has healing qualities and informs the gut-brain and vagus nerve of the plant's medicine, but if necessary add a small amount of honey or apple juice concentrate.

Cold infusions are used for herbs containing large amounts of mucilage, e.g., *Althea officinalis* marshmallow, linseed, psyllium. Aromatic herbs, those containing significant amounts of essential oil, are sometimes also extracted by cold infusion; soaking in cold water for 12 hours, this can be good if a cooling effect is being sought; for example, making cold *Tilia* or linden blossom infusion to calm hot flushes.

Teas can be prepared from a single species, or you can experiment with blending herbs together in a tea; there are some examples in the profiles, but this can be an extremely creative process and encourages us to work with taste, smell and the appearance of the tea.

Decoctions

Decoctions are used to prepare harder plant parts such as roots, barks, twigs, berries and seeds that need a stronger extraction method. Decocting is simply simmering in boiling water. The plant material, whether fresh or dried, should be cut or broken into small pieces before simmering to allow maximum extraction. The herbs are placed in a pan, covered with cold water and brought to the boil. They are then simmered for 20–30 minutes. In Chinese herbal practice, the herbs are traditionally decocted until the water volume is reduced by two-thirds, whilst in European herbal medicine the tradition is to reduce by one-third for internal use, and two-thirds for external use.

Use 20 g dried herbs or 40 g fresh herb in 750 ml cold water, reduced to about 500 ml by simmering, which is sufficient for 3–4 doses. The standard dose is 3–4 cups per day (about 500 ml), and decoctions may be stored in a similar way to infusions.

People often think that tinctures or capsules must be stronger than teas or decoctions, but this is not the case. Teas are extremely effective, and often the only impediment to using them is that people perceive their preparation as taking a lot of time. It does not really and the time that it takes for the kettle to boil and the tea to steep is often a good opportunity for a few minutes downtime which is sorely needed by a lot of people. Another approach is to make the day's supply of tea in a litre thermos flask to be drunk throughout the day. Comparing notes with colleagues and students, more and more of us are finding that teas are one of the most effective ways to give herbs. They are also cheaper and can be more sustainable; both considerations are becoming more important for many people.

Alcohol tinctures

Alcohol tinctures are made by soaking, or macerating, the herb in a mixture of alcohol and water for several weeks to dissolve the active constituents. The alcohol facilitates the extraction and also preserves the plant extract for up to 5 years. To prepare them you need a wine press or very strong hands. Normally one part of herb is added to five parts alcohol if dried herb is used, or one part to two for fresh herbs, but there are some exceptions to these rules and there are as many approaches to tincture making as there are people doing it. Judith Hoad, a traditional herbalist from Donegal, just packs her tincturing jars with herb material and pours over enough vodka to cover them before leaving to macerate whilst other people do very exact measuring of factors such as the water content of the herb, the precise percentage of alcohol needed and make the whole process extremely scientific or alchemic—it depends what floats your boat.

For those who wish to be a little more precise, the percentage strength of the alcohol solution depends on the plant being extracted, and it's constituents; for example, if resins are the main constituents (*Commiphora molmol*, myrrh) then 90% is used, if volatile oils are the main constituents 45% is used and if water-soluble constituents are the ones being extracted then 25% is used; having said this, in Ireland, the strongest proof alcohol the ordinary consumer can purchase is 40%, so many people just work with that.

Some people have developed a whole new creative art around tincturing; for example, Joe Nasr uses infusing or decocting or the preparation of aromatic waters as the first step in tincturing and believes that heat potentiates the process.

Probably the best starting place is to use 1:5 parts of dried herb or 1:2 of fresh, use 25% alcohol for plants that contain mainly water-soluble constituents and 40% for those requiring more alcohol for extraction. From that starting point, you can become as creative as you want to; it is all supposed to be fun, creative and a conversation with the process.

In Europe, the maximum dose used for most tinctures is 5 ml 2–3 times per day, but some have a substantially lower dose rate so double check this for any species that you are working with. Also, often a much lower dose is all that is needed, so start small and work up if in doubt. The plants give generously of their medicine, but we use them with healthy sustainable frugality in honour of their generosity.

Some books suggest that if one wishes to remove the alcohol from the tincture dose, it can be added to a small wineglassful of boiling water and left to stand for 5 minutes. Unfortunately, this will also remove any volatile compounds and does not remove much of the alcohol either. If alcohol is to be avoided, then it is better to use an alternative preparation, such as an infusion, decoction, vinegar tincture, aromatic water, capsule or juice.

Syrups

Syrups are sometimes prepared as a way of disguising unpalatable herbs for children (of all ages), as a way of preserving herbs, and are particularly useful for sore throats and coughs. Add 500 g of honey, sugar or apple juice concentrate to 500 ml of prepared infusion or decoction (1 ml of herbal extract to 1 g sweetener). The liquid and sweetener are then gently heated together until the sweetener is dissolved and the consistency is syrupy. The mixture is removed from the heat and cooled. The syrup can then be stored in sterilised jars or bottles with corks. Be aware that they do sometimes ferment and explode, so store with caution! They can be stored for about six months (preferably in the fridge), and the standard dose is 5–10 ml, three times a day. Two classics are elderberry syrup to boost the immune system, and as a gentle laxative at higher doses, and thyme/liquorice as a cough remedy. Syrups can also be used as cordial drinks in the winter and used as a food poured over ice cream, stewed fruit, fruit pies and crumbles and other foods.

Honeys

There are two kinds of herbal honeys.

The first type is honey made from a single species of plant by the bees; for example, one can sometimes obtain lavender or rosemary honey from France and other Mediterranean countries and lime blossom honey from Romania.

The other form is an infusion of herbs in honey. Two we make regularly are garlic honey which is a combination of mashed garlic with honey (one packs a jar with one- to two-thirds mashed garlic and then covers it with honey). This can also have some thyme or oregano added and is excellent for staving off the first signs of a cold or flu, just add a teaspoon to a cup of hot water and drink. It is also excellent spread on toast, added to stir-fries or salad dressings.

The second one is made by slicing an organic unwaxed lemon, packing it into a jar with some slivers of fresh ginger, covering with honey and leaving overnight. We often combine this one 2:1 with *Inula*, pine or elderflower vinegar to make an oxymel for treating coughs and colds. There are many herbs one can prepare in this way, and we prefer this to making glycerites; it is just as sticky but uses a local, unprocessed base and supports our local beekeepers and bees.

Herbal vinegars/vinegar tinctures/aceta

Although alcohol tinctures have predominated for the last century or so, we are finding that vinegar tinctures are a really good alternative. Some people find the sour taste a little challenging at first, but this really tones up the digestion and can help with heat in the digestive system. Vinegar is also better at extracting minerals from the herbs and helps with their absorption, especially calcium absorption, so these tinctures are particularly useful for bone repair, nerve function and have many other uses. Vinegar is also traditionally used to extract herbs high in alkaloids.

Vinegar tinctures can be taken internally in the same way as alcohol tinctures, individually or in blends. Some practitioners find that patient compliance (getting people to take them) can be an issue as a lot of people find the sourness challenging initially. They are really good when people wish to avoid alcohol. They can be mixed into a little fruit juice to help with taking them. They can also be sprinkled over vegetables, rice or salads as a food-medicine. In France, these vinegars are used as summer cordials due to their wonderfully cooling properties.

They are also excellent for the skin, treating inflammation, correcting the pH of the acid mantle and encouraging a good skin flora (most of our skin flora prefer an acid environment and overuse of soaps and detergents over alkalises the skin). They can be combined into creams or used in compresses and poultices. Added to drawing poultices, they potentise the action.

Paul Bergner says that William Cook, a Physiomedicalist of the 1800s, preferred vinegar as a menstruum for issues of the respiratory system. He felt that it concentrated the herb's actions to the respiratory system. And we have found this to be the case in practice.

They are really helpful in anti-inflammatory creams since the vinegar is also good at reducing inflammation.

Pickled herbs are another possibility—sushi ginger and many other possibilities. When we made our burdock vinegar we took a little of the pickled roots that had not been pressed off and added them to our forage salad; they were delicious. Other favourites are blackcurrant leaves and fennel seeds.

The classic weights and measures are:

* 200 g dried herb or 300 g fresh herb, finely chopped
* 1 litre organic cider vinegar

We have found that for dried leaves and flowers this approximates to loosely packing the jar and pouring over the vinegar. For dried barks, seeds, fruits and roots it approximates to packing the jar one-third full and covering with vinegar. For fresh material we just pack the jar a little tighter and pour in the vinegar.

The herbs are placed into a clean jar (sterilise with boiling water, Milton fluid, in a baby bottle steriliser or a microwave). Pour on the vinegar, ensuring that the herb is covered. Close the jar tightly and label with the date and contents. Shake thoroughly for 1–2 minutes to ensure that the herb is thoroughly soaked in the vinegar. Shake every day for 1–2 minutes for 14 days.

The easiest way to extract the vinegar is by using a wine press. Pour the mixture into the press and collect the liquids in a jug. Press down the material until no more can be extracted. If you do not have a wine press, strain the material through a jelly bag or muslin bag, then squeeze thoroughly, wearing food preparation gloves to prevent contamination. For small quantities, one can use a potato ricer lined with muslin to press off the vinegar.

Pour the pressed vinegar into sterilised jars or bottles and close firmly. Label the bottles clearly with the date and name of the preparation. Vinegars should keep for up to 3 years if stored in a cool, dark place. They can be used medicinally, to flavour food, as hair and skin tonics and as cleaning products (e.g. mopping floors, cleaning glass). For medicinal use, the standard dose is 5 ml three times daily in a little water or fruit juice for a healthy adult. Some people claim that this method is no good for extracting essential oil rich herbs, but I have not found that to be the case.

Live vinegars are a valuable fermented food that helps to alkalise the body, encourages good liver health and also tones the whole digestive system, including the pancreas and its secretions. Vinegars can help with the absorption of minerals and can act as a prebiotic that will encourage a healthy bowel flora. They have many uses both internally and topically.

As with all foods and fermentations local is best so in Ireland we would consider making apple cider vinegar as a first choice but you could also prepare malt vinegars from beer and other vinegars from hedgerow wines. The scope is very wide. Colleagues living in France use local wine vinegar since that is the local live variety.

Oxymels

An oxymel is basically a combination of vinegar and honey. The simplest version is to mix four parts honey with one part of apple cider vinegar or other vinegar. A more complex version is to mix one part water, one part vinegar and two parts of honey then simmer down to a third of the volume and then skim off any scum. Oxymels are a traditional folk medicine panacea, but used particularly for fevers, as a gargle for sore throats, to clear excess phlegm, for arthritis, gout, to promote weight loss (as a metabolic stimulant) and to promote longevity. They are diluted in water as a refreshing drink as well. Obviously, one can use aromatic honeys (ones from particular species, or ones with essential oil incorporated) or vinegar tinctures to enhance the therapeutic effect.

Metheglins and meads

Traditional mead is a natural ferment similar to a wine made with honey water and yeast. It is usually made using wild yeasts although it is possible to get cultured yeast from home brewing suppliers.

There are quite a few variations on this such as:

- Braggot is mead made with malted grains
- A rhodomel is made with rose petals
- A pyment is made with grapes/grape juice
- Cyser is made with apples
- A melomel is made with fruit or berries
- Capsicumel is made with chillis and assorted peppers
- Bochet is made with caramelised honey to give a deeper flavour
- Hydromels are made with less honey

- Sack is made with more honey
- A metheglin is made with a spice or herb infusion rather than just plain water
- And an acerglyn is made substituting maple syrup for the honey

Over a period of time, the yeasts acclimatise to being fed with honey, so if one varies the source of saccharides (from honey, to honey combined with fruit juice or maple syrup) the yeast may need an adaptation period but then it gets into full swing again.

Mead is probably the oldest fermented alcoholic drink known to humans. It is not just a recreational drink though; it has been shown to have great health benefits which can be enhanced by including herbs, berries and spices.

Mead contains antioxidants and other compounds with health benefits from the honey used. Recent research has shown that chrysin, a flavonoid found in abundance in honey, has the ability to inhibit the proliferation of and induce apoptosis (cell death) in cancer cells and also suppresses neuroinflammation.

Olofsson, a Swedish research scientist, has studied 'lactic acid bacteria', or LABs, that live inside the honeybee's crop, a special stomach devoted to nectar collection. These bacteria exude a mixture of antimicrobial compounds that target and kill pathogens. When honey is inoculated with LABs, it can be used to treat chronic, antibiotic-resistant wounds in horses and has been shown to eliminate human pathogens, including the notoriously drug-resistant MSRA in vitro.

Unpasteurised wild honey mead contains all 13 LABs and wild yeasts that ferment mead spontaneously (method below). Pasteurised and intensively produced honey does not contain all these bacteria. And commercial mead normally uses a strain of wine yeast rather than wild yeast and uses a sterilised honey and water mixture, eliminating the possibility of any of the wild yeast strains being present.

Our starter mead recipe was adapted from a Galloway Wild Foods website post:

Take a jar of unpasteurised honey (although we have used pasteurised local honey and organic honey to good effect too).

A 454 g jar of honey represents 22,700 bee trips (at 0.02 g pollen per trip), so it is precious stuff indeed.

Ideally, use spring water or well water or mineral water. However, we have tended to use boiled and cooled tap water left to stand to evaporate the chlorine off. Our tap water is fairly hard, but the mead does not seem to mind.

Mix the honey into about five times the volume of water (2.5 litres per jar); this is easier to do if you warm the water to tepid. Use a glass vessel, either use a larger kilner jar or a pyrex bowl covered in a tea towel or muslin. At this dilution, you can expect a full fermentation cycle to yield a drink of 10–15% alcohol. If you want a lower alcohol content, you can stop the fermentation earlier and end up with an effervescent beverage.

Stir or shake the mixture daily, preferably using a wooden spoon. After about three days, a frothy head forms and a cloudy yeast deposit also forms. I tend to cover in between stirring to keep things out, and the yeasts still seem to colonise happily, but you can leave the vessel open if you wish. If using a kilner only cover with muslin since otherwise too much pressure builds up.

The fermentation process can take up to a week to establish at room temperature.

A shorter fermentation yields a sweeter drink with more bubbles and less alcohol (after a week or two), or you can leave it for 4–6 weeks for a drier and more alcoholic drink.

At that point, the mead can be syphoned into bottles for storage or racked off into a demijohn to clear before bottling. Some people recommend ageing mead for up to 5 years, but we have only managed to keep some for a year.

When you syphon off the beverage, you can retain the wild yeasts and use them to start new batches or to experiment with some of the related beverages such as metheglins, pyments and so forth. If you do not want to use it immediately, it can be stored in the fridge for a few weeks.

If you are using the saved yeast culture, make a solution of honey to fill a demijohn, or dissolve the honey and make up the volume with a herb tea or fruit juice. Add the yeast starter, put in an airlock and leave to ferment until completed (no more burps through the airlock). Rack off into a clean demijohn, leaving the yeast slug behind (which makes the new starter) and after a week or so bottle. It should be great medicine for the stomach and gut flora and be full of B vitamins as a live ferment.

For a metheglin, one can use either hot or cold infusion. I have only tried the hot method.

The cold infusion method means just adding whatever herb you fancy to mead whilst it ferments.

The hot infusion method requires making an infusion or decoction of your chosen plants. This is then left to cool, before mixing with the honey and fermenting as above.

Always strain out any residual plant matter before bottling.

We have found that the meads are wonderfully therapeutic—sour cherry or bilberry for sleep, Angelica for digestion, bitter combo for toning the liver and gut-brain, rose for calming, rosehip or pine for coughs, elderberry for flus.

Poultices

Poultices are made with a mixture of fresh, dried or powdered herbs, simmered or simply steeped in the minimum quantity of water for two minutes and applied externally. Marshmallow root powder, green clay, or linseed can be added to give a better texture and for their own drawing qualities, especially for infected wounds, ulcers or boils. Poultices are also used for nerve and muscle pain, sprains and broken bones—in these cases a small pinch of ginger or a couple of drops of ginger oil may be added to 'potentise' the action. Poultices may also be used for mastitis or engorged breasts—either cold cabbage leaves or warm calendula. Try to ensure that only sufficient water is present when simmering or soaking in hot water to form a firm texture without having to squeeze off any liquid; apply some oil to the area being treated to prevent the poultice sticking; the herbs are applied as hot as possible, taking care not to scald the skin. The herbs are laid on lint and covered with gauze, then the poultice is applied gauze side to skin and bandaged in place. It may be left for between 30 minutes and 24 hours, depending on what is being treated.

Compresses

Compresses are the application of a soft cloth or clean flannel/towel, soaked in an appropriate infusion, decoction or diluted tincture, either hot or cold, depending on what is being treated.

Powders

Powders are an alternative to the liquid forms for internal use and can also be used in external preparations. Once a herb is powdered, it is more susceptible to oxidation due to the fact that a larger surface area is exposed to the air. This means that powders need to be kept in airtight containers and used before they lose their potency. Powders are a great way to use herbs for adding into food; they can be sprinkled on soups or other foods, added to smoothies or used to prepare infusions. They can also be used to pack capsules. Capsule fillers are available from various sources online. Capsules suitable for vegans and vegetarians are also available from several suppliers. The standard dose is 2–3 00 size capsules twice a day—this dose contains about 250 mg of herb. The equivalent amount of powdered herb could also be sprinkled on food, or mixed into a stiff dough with honey (2 parts powder to 1 part honey) rolled out into a sausage about the width of the little finger, cut into segments and rolled into pills that can be stored in the fridge; we find patient compliance excellent with these. Vegans can use glycerin instead of honey. Powders are also used in some external preparations, such as poultices, ointments and creams; these forms of preparations are described below.

Aromatic waters

Aromatic waters are also known as hydrosols, hydrolats, distillates, floral waters or flower waters. They are the water phase of steam distillation, saturated with water-soluble volatile components such as alcohols and acids. These have their own therapeutic properties and are widely used in continental Europe. Aromatic waters can also be prepared from plants with little or no essential oil content; in France and other countries on the continent, many rural households will have a small still for preparing this sort of medicine to use at home. Hydrosols are used internally at a similar standard dose as that of tinctures; they can also be used externally as skin washes, and as ingredients in creams or compresses. They are also used in cooking.

N.B. mixing distilled water and essential oils does not produce the same product. For home use, aromatic waters can be prepared using a pressure cooker or a preserving pan.

Macerated or infused oils

Macerated or infused oils are made by soaking the herb in cold-pressed unrefined vegetable oil (almond, olive, sunflower are commonly used) for several weeks to obtain a cold infusion or by gently heating to about 60°C over a water bath for about three hours for a hot infusion. Once the maceration process is complete, the oil is put through a press to complete the extraction and remove the spent herb. This process extracts the fat-soluble components of the herb for use in massage oils, liniments, creams and ointments. If a stronger preparation is required, then the process is sometimes repeated with a fresh batch of herb. They will keep for up to a year if stored in a cool, dry place.

Hot method

1. 250 g dried or 500 g fresh herb.
2. 750 ml cold pressed virgin and preferably organic vegetable oil (olive oil is the most stable for heating).
3. Mix the chopped herbs and oil together in a pyrex bowl and place over a pan of boiling water. Cover and simmer gently for 2–3 hours.
4. Remove from the heat and allow to cool, then pour into a wine press as described for the vinegars, or through a muslin bag.
5. Collect the strained oil in a sterile jug and pour into sterile bottles— label with date and contents.
6. Store in a cool dark place for up to 1 year.

Cold method

1. Loosely pack a sterile jar with fresh or dried herb. Herbs with a high water content such as calendula, chickweed, basil or comfrey are best prepared with dried herb, or by the hot method to prevent them from going rancid. St. John's wort is best prepared by the cold method.
2. Place the jar on a sunny windowsill or in the hot press and leave for 2–6 weeks.
3. Strain as described for vinegars.
4. Label and stored as described above.

Infused oils may be used for culinary purposes, as massage oils or as the base to prepare ointments and creams.

Ointments/salves/balms

Ointments/salves/balms are oil-based mixtures that help to protect the skin and only contain oily ingredients. They can be thickened with any wax, including paraffin wax, but beeswax is preferable as it has its own therapeutic proprieties. Use unbleached beeswax. If beeswax is not available use cocoa butter or another plant wax/or fat. Previously, duck or goose fat and pig lard have been used and would be deemed to have their own therapeutic benefits. Ointments stay on the skin for a long time, so they are useful for forming barriers to protect the skin. They are also healing and soothing. They are good for nappy rash, and for protecting the lips. They are also useful for dry areas such as knees, heels, feet and elbows. They also keep heat and water in so they are good for rheumatic aches, dehydrated skin and conditions made worse by cold weather. Do not use them if the skin is hot, inflamed or weepy.

- 300 ml infused oil or base oil.
- 25 g beeswax; shredded or in beads.

Warm the ingredients together in a bain-marie just to the point where the waxes melt. Add essential oils if desired and pour into clean jars. Label and leave to set in the fridge.

Plaisters are made by spreading the ointment onto clean bandage. Cover the bandage with a layer of oilcloth and roll up to store. Place in an airtight container in the fridge, or a cool, dry place. Label with the ingredients and date. They are a convenient way of applying ointment to aching joints etc. All these preparations should be used within 9–12 months.

Creams

Creams are lighter than ointments as they contain water and oil in an emulsion. Creams are more cooling than ointments and are absorbed more quickly. They are more suitable for hot, inflamed and weepy skin conditions. They are also useful for applying to warm areas of the body such as the groin. The ones described below are water in oil emulsions, which are good for moisturising. Oil in water emulsions are more difficult to make at home. A basic cream can be made with:

- 50 ml of oil
- 15 g beeswax
- 50 ml water/infusion/decoction/floral water/tincture

Cream method: make sure ingredients are weighed accurately on a clean scale; otherwise consistency will be affected. If beeswax is being used then shred finely before weighing or use beads. Put oily and fatty ingredients into a stainless steel or pyrex bowl (oils, beeswax, cocoa butter etc.). Put watery ingredients—floral waters, spring water, decoction, infusion or tincture—into a separate stainless steel or pyrex bowl and stand both bowls in a shallow pan of water or bain-marie over a gentle heat. Liquid lecithin can be added to the oily ingredients to help emulsification; borax can be added to the watery ingredients for the same effect. Stir the bowl with the fatty ingredients to facilitate melting, remove both bowls from the heat. The best way to form an emulsion is to use an electric egg beater or blender wand on its lowest speed. Alternatively, use an egg whisk or a balloon whisk. Add the water slowly (a few drops at a time, increasing to a small stream), until it is all incorporated—like making mayonnaise. When all the water has been added stop beating at once, too much beating can make the cream separate. If adding essential oils, stir in carefully. The cream can then be put into jars and left in the fridge until set. Make sure to label jars with ingredients and date. The cream can also be divided into several jars and different essential oils added to the individual jars.

The formulae can be multiplied up to make larger batches of cream. Once the technique has been mastered, you can also play around with the proportions to make lighter or firmer creams—enjoy.

To increase the shelf life, part of the oily ingredients can be substituted with wheat germ oil, or with vitamin E oil. The base oil can also be varied to give a different quality of cream. Essential oils that are particularly good for preserving the creams are lavender, tea tree or benzoin. None of these are as effective as the preservatives that are used in commercial creams, but they will give a longer shelf life. Storing in the fridge will also lengthen shelf life. Also, rather than dipping fingers into the jars using a spatula or spoon to dispense the cream.

Before making any of these preparations, you need to prepare your equipment and ensure that it is spotlessly clean. Use stainless steel, or glass containers, bowls and pans. Use stainless steel implements, for stirring, mixing, chopping ingredients and so on.

Avoid using any dirty jars, or implements, tie back long hair and keep fingers out of all mixtures to prevent contamination. Any preparations that show signs of contamination (mould growing or smelling 'off') should be discarded immediately. Occasionally, water will 'bleed' out of the cream. This does not mean that they have gone off, but that some separation has occurred. They are still ok to use.

Incense

Incense have been used for thousands of years. The preparation of blends of aromatic plants to be used in healing (as simple as fumigating to prevent disease or for more complex reasons) and for spiritual practice and ritual is a beautiful art.

Blends may be created for a specific ceremony (births, birthdays, weddings, funerals), for rituals—to clear the space, create a sacred space, to aid prayer and meditation, for fumigation of houses or animal housing, for the treatment of maladies (physical, emotional or spiritual) and for the pure pleasure of perfuming a space. Incense was traditionally used outside or in large communal places or worship so the traditional preparations can be a little overwhelming in a small space and can create a lot of smoke (beware of setting off fire alarms).

Ingredients used can include: resins; aromatic woods (many of these have become endangered, so you may wish to replace with native species such as willow and oak); spices; dried leaves and flowers; essential oils; raisins soaked in wine; beeswax; there are a huge variety of possible ingredients (for example cocoa powder adds a seriously delicious note).

Equipment: pestle and mortar, or coffee grinder, for herbs and spices labels and storage jars.

Quite simply, you assemble your chosen ingredients, grind them and blend them together then place in a jar. It is better to allow the ingredients to meld and mature together for at least seven days before using, as a sort of 'alchemic' process occurs between the ingredients.

Smudge smoke and fumigation

In this part of the world, we mislaid some of our traditions (we did not lose them, we just forgot where we put them) and so we have looked to our neighbours in other parts of the world to remind us of them.

Much of the way in which smudging and smoking is practised in this part of the world now is borrowed from the Native American traditions, and the most widely used plant at present tends to be white sage or sage-brush (*Artemisia tridentata/ludoviciana*) which is native to Northern America. In this tradition, smudging sticks and herbs were never sold but rather given as gifts and yet most of the white sage we use in this part of the world does not respect this part of their tradition, and therefore it seems more appropriate to look to our own plants, rather than encourage the appropriation and disrespect of commercialising the American tradition.

In most cultures throughout the world, smoke, smudge and incense would have formed part of ritual and ritual was seen as part of the sacred ordinary and ordinary sacredness; bear in mind that many of these rituals had a practical reason too, so smudging and smoking was not just about removing spiritual contamination but was protected against airborne disease and helped clear ticks, lice and other little bugs from the fur and hair of people and animals. In most places there was no clear distinction between medicine and spirituality; the priest(ess)/healer-doctor would have looked after people's physical, emotional and spiritual health in the community. So smoke was used as an offering to the deities and the sacred, for meditation and ritual, but also to cleanse animals (including the human ones) and make them healthy; for fumigation and space clearing; to preserve food and in some places squatting over smoke was used cleanse and repair the womb after childbirth.

The amount of ritual and complexity for preparation of plants for smoking varied from place to place; in ancient Egypt, there were very complex recipes and formulae for creating incenses, as there continue to be in places such as India, Nepal and Japan where burning incense is seen as an important part of spiritual rituals.

Amongst the European peasant cultures smokes and smudges often had more practical applications in the sacred ordinary to ensure the clearing of parasites and bugs from domestic animals and to clear 'bad air'. Fumigation by smoke would also have been performed as a medicinal practice. In France, rosemary and thyme were burned in hospitals as a way of keeping the air clean and preventing contagion. Chris Hedley and Non Shaw, in their excellent book *Herbal Remedies*, describe how smoking mixtures were widely used for the treatment of asthma and respiratory problems by burning on charcoal or using pipes or rolled into cigarettes until relatively recently. Smoking with herbs was deemed to relax a tight chest and relieve night wheezes and asthma. The herbs would be sprinkled on charcoal or onto a fire or barbecue.

In this part of the world plants that were traditionally used in smoke purification included vervain, mugwort, pine and juniper. Often herbs were dried as loose leaf and burned on charcoal or thrown onto fires; vervain and mugwort work better dried as loose leaves. For pine and juniper small branchlets can be dried and used as smudge sticks. Rosemary also works well this way.

To make smudge bundles, one of the best herbs to use is garden sage (*Salvia officinalis*) although other herbs such as thyme, lavender and mugwort can be included in the bundles. To tie the bundles, use cotton; nettle fibre or couch grass strands have also been used to good effect by one of the students here. I often tie bundles with natural garden twine which is then removed before lighting the bundle.

You may choose to grow particular plants in your garden specifically to use for smudge or to collect them from the wild. Before harvesting set your intention and sit a whilst with the plant to ask permission to harvest part of it and use it for this purpose. Often people will leave an offering for the plant—tobacco, corn, a hair from their head or a simple prayer of thanksgiving. Make sure to harvest respectfully not taking too much of the plant. Use strong, healthy plant material. Some people use a particular number of sprigs tied together depending on the significance of the number for themselves. You may choose to wilt the herbs for a day before tying them or simply tie them fresh. Hold the herbs in a tight bundle then, using your chosen binding, wrap it tightly around in a spiral weave. Tuck the top leaves over and bind them closely then bind back down the smudge stick and tie a knot. I tend to dry the smudge sticks in the hot press (airing cupboard) to ensure that they are thoroughly dried the whole way through so that they do not go mouldy; this takes a few weeks. I prefer a simple ritual prayer to be offered before harvesting and tying the bundles: give thanks to the plants and the Earth for the abundance around us, take a moment to clear the heart and work from pure innocent intention and if the smudge is being used for clearing a group space ask that it will be good medicine for this, or if it is to be used personally put this into the intention. If one feels that the plant does not wish to be used, then do not harvest it; if one's energy does not feel in tune with the harvesting and tying, leave it to another person or another time. And remember to give thanks after harvesting and whilst making the bundles, gratitude is a great balm. And remember to say a prayer of intention before smudging too.

Here are some brief notes on a few that we use.

- Juniper is calming, protective and clears out negative energy. It also helps ward off viral infections and airborne illness. It can be grown easily.
- Pine is grounding, cleansing, purifying and helps to bring forgiveness. It helps to deepen the breathing and clear phlegm and strengthen the adrenal glands. Our native pine is a tall tree, but one can grow smaller varieties of pine or spruce in the garden in containers.
- Mugwort is a native plant, and its scientific name is *Artemisia vulgaris*. It is considered to be a messenger plant, helping us connect with Nature, protective and helping lucid dreaming. It is especially cleansing and used to treat parasites and for menstrual imbalance and is a wayside journeying plant.
- Vervain is a native plant that is used for balance, repairing fragmentation, inner strength and peace. It is a tonifying nervine which works on the liver and heart and digestion.
- Bay is not a native, but many people grow it in their garden. It is seen as a guardian plant that wards of illness and is traditionally used to make wreaths for champions.
- Sage is not a native but grows really well in our climate. It is associated with clearing, cleansing, fertility, healing, wisdom, mental clarity and longevity.
- Rosemary is not a native either and needs to be planted in dry soil. It also strengthens the memory, helps with energy flow, binds the soul into the body, promotes fidelity and protects space. It also protects against airborne pathogens.
- Thyme protects against airborne pathogens too and is often combined with rosemary. It promotes courage and confidence and lifts heavy moods, bringing an increase in energy and vitality.

Other plants that we have found valuable are wood betony, myrtle and lavender and you may well find yourself drawn to use others since the plant allies are so very giving and generous.

Flower essences

Flower essences are another form that can be prepared in many ways. The traditional way is to sit with the plant and listen to what its medicine is and then take a flower/leaf/fruit and place it in a bowl of spring water in the sun for several hours in an undisturbed place. The plant material is then removed with twigs or chopsticks, and the water is preserved by adding a spirituous liquid (vodka/brandy/eau de vie/ whisky) to it. Cathy Skipper adds one-third of spirit to two-thirds of water when making these preparations in the Beaujolais region, but I tend to use two-thirds spirit to one-third water due to the high humidity in Ireland. We also have a challenge of getting several hours of sunlight here so sometimes it is necessary to adapt the method by placing the water and flowers into a closed jar, and placing it for several hours outside in whatever weather prevails. Moon essences can be made at night by the light of the moon. It is generally felt that it is ok to pick the flowers by hand but avoid putting fingers into the water. One can also use a hot method if there is no sun, placing the bowl into a bain-marie. Some people do not place the plant material into the water; they sit with the plant and then just focus intention into the water; this method has been used to prepare animal essences and flower essences.

Once the mother essence has been prepared, it is taken through a series of dilutions to make the dispensing bottle given to the client. Add 7 (or 1 or whatever number intuitively feels right) drops of mother essence to a 30 ml dropper bottle of brandy or other spirit to make a stock bottle. Use the same number of drops of stock bottle added to a 30 ml dropper bottle of brandy, apple cider vinegar, aromatic water or spring water to make a dispensing bottle to give to a client with instructions to use 2–7 drops in a bottle of water to sip during the day, or 1–2 drops under the tongue or on pulse points as required. The essence can also be added to tincture formulae or skin creams or perfumes.

Baths

Bathing with herbs has a long tradition. In Ireland, there are still several places that offer seaweed baths for health. Herbal baths can be used for many purposes. Footbaths are really good for detoxifying the system and stimulating the circulation. Hand baths can be valuable for arthritic hands. Full body baths can be great for delivering a good dose of herbs transdermally (through the skin). Our skin is permeable to many of the plants' constituents, and they get straight into the general circulation. Sitz baths are used to treat the bowel, kidneys, reproductive organs and congestion in the abdomen and pelvis and problems with the hips. For a sitz bath one needs two containers that are large enough to sit in; one contains hot water with the herbs or oils added, the other contains cool water. One sits first in the hot water and herbs with the feet in the cool water so that the circulation and the medicine are drawn into the lower trunk for about 10 minutes. Then one sits in the cool water with the feet in the hot water for 10 minutes to draw the circulation to the extremities. This can be repeated several times. Baths can be prepared with infusions, decoctions or essential oils and salt or Epsom salts may also be used.

There are many other forms in which herbs can be used; these ones are easy enough to prepare and fun to make at home.

PART III

THE HUMAN PLANT

This part of the book shifts our focus onto the human, the human condition and health. We combine a blend of metaphysics, old traditional insights and cutting-edge science to give us insights into ourselves and how plants can help to bring us into healthy alignment.

CHAPTER SEVEN

Community, connection and boundaries

Note: when exploring the human condition, it is helpful to remember that we are human beings and therefore this is an exploration of who we are. As you read and study, it can be helpful to meditate upon the knowledge bringing it into your own being as an understanding of who you are.

We live in a constant conversation that is as old as the world. Humans were once aware of this every minute of each day and knew how to tap into the constant stream of communication that flows through the natural world physically, emotionally, mentally, spiritually.

Communities were egalitarian, bio-centred, matrifocal and based on equity. There was no hierarchy or dominator, and the community centred partnership included all the community of Nature, not just the anthropocentric, economic, ownership-based epistemology that we follow now.

Then a rather large epistemological mistake shifted our centre of perception from our hearts and our guts up to our heads, and specifically our neo-cortex. Along with this shift came ideas about domination, ownership and capitalism. Our hearts and minds were colonised with false ideas about being separate from the rest of the beings that inhabit this planet alongside us. We began to view ourselves as separate from our kin of other species, then from members of our own species (racism, sexism, ageism, classism), until we reached the point of seeing ourselves as so separate from Nature that even our own bodies may seem alien. The external wounds started appearing, as the natural world became nothing more than resources to plunder and deplete. Rather than gathering enough from the generous abundance that this planet affords us the idea of ownership and profit came into being. Profit, accumulation and capital gain were needed; an underclass was needed, and competition for the top of the heap became a concept that was laudable. Now we need to a return to a more natural way of being in the world and remembering what the true nature and ecological function of a human being is; our survival as a species depends on this, and so does the survival of much of life on Earth.

Returning to our true nature is simple; we step into what we were born to do. Anyone can do it; it is not just for a few chosen people or people with special gifts; anyone who says that it is not for ordinary people is telling a lie. We are all ordinary human beings with the ability to gather information from the heart of the world; we are all able to perceive the meanings of things because this is part of our natural native ability. Often professional groupings will create a complicated vocabulary around their work in order to keep it for themselves, in order to be exclusive, to exclude others from part of our common heritage. We see it happening amongst some groups that we might not expect it to such as those involved in ecology, the green movement, complementary health care.

We are being fed a lot of lies about our food, our medicine, our place in the world, economics, about the balance of power. Most of the things that really matter are not grandiose and should not be costly or complicated: water, food, shelter, sunlight, warmth, love, companionship, hugs, smiles, tears. They can be hard work; being real is hard work as it is not sophisticated (lost in sophistry) or glamorous (lost in or covered by illusion).

When we inhabit the world in which we walk without illusion, then we can step onto our path and know who we truly are. Actually, life is more about re-discovering every moment who we are and why we are here; we can make that connection into spirit which allows us to do that and we can make the connections that allow us to recognise that we are part of the web rather than trying to stand outside our ecological niche.

We step into integrity; being whole, with all the parts integrated. As we move towards integrity, we see that we are an integral part of the whole picture, of the scenario of the Universe. The connectedness of all things becomes apparent. We see that science and linear analytical thinking are not all that there is, nor are they superior to the other ways of describing the world. Science cannot answer all questions since its vocabulary only covers the linear approach, the dissection and analysis of the material world in a particular way. It is a valuable way of taking something apart and seeing what it is made of, but then we are no longer working with whole, living systems. Nature becomes non-living and not conscious; something is lost—the vitality is gone.

It's like this—give a group of toddlers a big pile of building blocks of all shapes and colours. They might decide to put all the red ones together, or all the cubes together, all the blues ones in one pile, or all the pyramids in another heap—they have engaged in a linear analytical process of categorising and describing by reductionism. This is a good process. However, they do not stop there. After a whilst they will throw them all back together and start to build something—a castle, a dragon, a village, a forest, a space ship. They have employed analytical thought, linearity to see what the parts are, and then they move onto the next stage: engaging the right brain, creativity, consilience, combining science and art, spirit and material to create a whole picture (in this case one with three or more dimensions, as they may well inhabit what they have built with imaginary creatures, plants, characters which brings in several more dimensions).

Direct perception and gathering information by multidimensional sensing

When we reawaken our multiple senses turn on; we start to feel the world, taste it, hear it, smell it, see it with those senses that can sense the invisibles. We start to access knowledge, information and wisdom directly from the world. We perceive with our hearts, our guts and those senses that have been dulled by civilisation and domestication, by the perceived mechanisation of the Universe. We become connected to the visible and the invisible. It can feel quite strange and overwhelming, but it is safe. Being wild is much safer than being tamed. Wild does not mean out of control, it means authentically in the natural state. Living in the moment does not mean being irresponsible, it means fully engaging in the process of being present, conscious and aware of what we are doing and the possible futures it may create.

The plants help us to remember who we are.

An exercise listening to the stories of the earth

Take a moment to make sure that you are fully present in the place where you are sitting, leaving the cares and concerns of your everyday life to one side, outside the door. Allow your mind to relax; there is no hurry.

Take a moment to focus your breath into your heart. Take a few deep breaths and direct the energy of your breath into your heart space, allow your heart to relax, that is its natural state.

Remember a time when you were a young child, and you climbed onto the lap of some kind person that you loved and trusted completely, rested your head on their chest, against their heart, breathing each other in and out; feeling safe, feeling loved, feeling protected. And then you settled into listening to their voice telling you a magical story, leading you into a realm full of mystery and wonder; taking you on a journey to that place so vividly that you could see it, smell it, taste it, hear it, feel it and touch it.

Imagine now that you are sitting on the lap of the Earth and allow yourself to open up your senses to experiencing her stories, the stories she has been telling since the dawn of time, the stories we need to hear to remind us of who we are, to remember ourselves.

And, by the way, you can step into this place of receptivity and take that open perception with you as you go out to the plants to listen to their stories. You can also take that open perception with you as you meet the active constituents in the plant by tasting and smelling and using your senses to engage with the molecules in a cup of herbal tea or a tincture. We can investigate the scientific view of the world from this way of perceiving. They are not mutually exclusive; your inner botanist, your inner clinical herbalist, your inner research scientist can all engage in the process of meeting the plants, one complex being meeting with another.

Humans are ecosystems too

Western orthodox medical science has put a lot of time and effort into mapping the geography of the body and elucidating the processes that happen in health and disease, although it tends to concentrate on pathologising normal physiological states. It has relentlessly dissected our physicality down to its smallest minutiae in an attempt to explain the function of a machine. However, it is also important to realise that 'a rose cannot be described with a ruler'; we are part of Nature and Nature is not made up of straight lines. If only the linear, analytical approach is used in trying to understand our own bodies and our place in the ecosystem, we are left with a very narrow view. If we view the human organism as just the physical body, and the body purely as a machine to be fixed, or a stream of biochemical processes to be balanced, we are ignoring large parts of who we are.

We need to remember that non-linear, analogous thinking is a large part of our normal or natural mode of thinking; humans are a part of the ecosystem as a macrocosm, and each organism is a microcosmic ecosystem. It is the concept of the separation of humans from the natural web that causes problems because then we no longer realise or believe that we are part of the macrocosm, part of the community, part of the council of beings. If we see ourselves as separate, we can excuse exploitative, cruel behaviour.

The inner wounds in humans and the exterior wounds in the world occur as a result of this.

It is probable that there are no evolutionary accidents as regards the human design; so, as we start to map the human, we need to ask questions like why are the adrenal glands on top of the kidneys? And then we can find answers that satisfy us on all levels—physically, energetically, poetically, emotionally, spiritually. We all have different questions because we are each a unique individual; the human species is not a monoculture. We each have our own journey, and we each are called to find and live our own truth. We are also called to share our own truth, our own story in order to do the work of co-creating, reweaving the tapestry of our communal story; this is the magnum opus of the Universe.

All life on Earth shares a common ancestry: we all evolved from bacteria. This means that we have a common ancestry with all other life forms on the planet, including the plants. Furthermore, within the cells of all eukaryotes are organelles called mitochondria that have different DNA to the main cell, DNA that is solely inherited from the maternal line which provides the matter of the embryo. Plants also contain organelles called chloroplasts, or more properly plastids since there are also chromoplasts and amyloplasts; these plastids also contain different DNA to the main cell and are from the maternal line. The DNA in the organelles is more similar to that of the prokaryotes. It is thought that a symbiosis arose between the eukaryotic ancestor and the mitochondrial ancestors.

Eukaryotes have a more resilient cell wall and therefore offered protection to the mitochondrial ancestor; the payback for the eukaryotic ancestor for taking on a passenger was that mitochondria are excellent at producing energy from food sources. For plants, the advantage of accepting an additional type of passenger—the chloroplast—was that these were able to actually produce food from a combination of sunlight, water and carbon dioxide, relieving the cell of the energy-expensive necessity to move to sources of food. The main cell nucleus contains equal amounts of DNA from the mother and the father.

When we look at our cells, we discover several things:

Firstly, that bacteria are our ancestors. We have tended to be somewhat xenophobic towards them in recent times, focusing purely on the differences and ignoring the similarities. In fact, only 10–50% of a person is made up of human cells, depending on whom you listen to, with the rest being composed of micro-organisms that live in/on us as an ecosystem.

Secondly, animal and plant cells are not so very different; they are different regarding the structure of the cell wall and the large vacuoles of fluid that plant cells contain in order to maintain a rigid structure without a skeleton, but apart from this we are essentially very similar on a cellular level, both as regards the functioning organelles that the cells contain and the way that many biochemical processes occur within the cell.

Third, most of the matter (mater, material) of the embryo comes from the ovum, including the organelle genome and half the nuclear DNA; the sperm or pollen brings the other half of the nuclear DNA and the ability to merge with the egg to create new life. The main inheritance of our material form comes from our maternal ancestors.

Fourth, each cell is a very small ecosystem.

Ancestral timelines

Simple single cell prokaryotes probably emerged about 3.8 billion years ago. Some of these cells started to photosynthesise about 3 million years ago, and the first complex eukaryotic single cell organisms probably emerged about 2 billion years ago. It took another billion years for multi-cellular life forms to emerge. Land plants are thought to have existed for about 475 million years, developing seeds after another 75 million years and flowers after another 345 million years. After the emergence of the first simple animals it took significant amounts of time for arthropods to emerge, followed by complex animals which developed into fish, then insects, then amphibians, followed by reptiles, mammals and then birds. All the dinosaurs (except the ones that evolved into birds) died out about 65 million years ago. The *Homo* genus emerged about 2.5 million years ago, but we did not start looking like we do today until about 200,000 years ago and the *Neanderthals* died out about 25,000 years ago, although we still retain about 4% of their DNA within ourselves since there was interbreeding between the *Neanderthals* and other *Homo* ancestors.

Over time different forms emerged: arthropod, insect, arachnid, crustacean, fish, amphibian, plant, reptile, mammal. These diversified to fulfil different roles in various niches, either to compete with other forms or to form communities to support survival, depending on our own particular epistemology. Darwin tended to promote the competition theory of evolution with competition and aggression being the driving force of evolution; the capitalist model of divergence. Lamarck tended to support the idea that evolution was driven by community and cooperation, but this was not a popular epistemology at the time and therefore was not promoted as a theory that would support the political and social structures that were prevalent. However, the validity of Lamarck's work is being reconsidered as we are starting to shift our paradigm.

Each species has a quintessential form; studying these can give us clues to our true nature and to aspects of our ancestral inheritance.

For example, Plant gives rise to subclasses such as tree, fern, moss, herb. But they are all expressions of Plant. Within Tree we have the gymnosperms which do not have flowers and bear naked seeds and tend to produce less complex ranges of secondary metabolites, since they tend to be wind pollinated; and then angiosperms which produce flowers and may produce complex colour, or scent compounds in order to attract pollinators, or to entice various animals to eat their fruit to aid wide seed dispersal. Attracting pollinators can help facilitate a wider dispersal of pollen, giving a greater genetic diversity of progeny and therefore a higher likelihood of adaptation and survival.

Within angiosperms, we have families and genuses with certain characteristics in common. Then we can narrow down our understanding to that of a particular species. Let's take oak (*Quercus robur*). And then we get to the individual oak tree that expresses oakness according to its internal and external environment. Plants and animals can re-write their DNA depending on the environment in which they live and according to their internal environment too; genes are switched on and off depending on our response to the communications and meanings that we experience. This concept is called epigenetics. So, an oak tree that is growing at the top of a mountain with high UV radiation and lots of rain will look significantly different to one growing in a low land forest or one growing by itself in a field. A mugwort plant growing on Irish wasteland, or by an English motorway, will look amazingly different from one growing by the roadside in Italy or France. It will also smell and taste different.

Applying this idea to humans, we are mammals, primates, great apes (the nearest ape relative that we speciated from is the chimpanzee), hominids, and humans (*Homo sapiens sapiens*), and then we are the individual expression of human which adjusts to its internal environment, its physical environment, its emotional and mental environment and its spiritual environment. We can trace back as far as we like along the line of our heritage to give us more and more clues about who we are.

As we explore this more deeply, reaching back through time to the moment of the Big Bang, the conception of the Universe when the planets were born, we realise that in this massive release of energy the stars came into being; the planets and stars made up of the matter, the stardust that would eventually give rise to life. So, we are truly the children of the stars, we are stardust made from the earth, from dust and we still have starlight in our hearts.

We can look back along our heritage, extract meanings and begin to see what being a human truly is. We can also trace the moment of our conception to the present time in our lives to examine the influences that have encouraged us to develop the particular expression of humanity that we are. In both instances, we can also realise that we have a choice regarding those internal genetic blueprints that we possess, how we choose to express them in the world and how we choose to react to our internal and external environments. Yes, this is within a certain set of parameters—we are human, not oak, not dolphin. However, as well as being human, we are all born with harmonies inside us that may be the shape of all manner of things; stone, oak, rose, tree, bear, and we can decide to identify these and fill them with whatever makes us whole. Or we can decide not to look beneath the surface, not to engage in rigorous self-examination to find deeper and deeper meanings. We can choose to stay on the surface, applying the linear mind, analysing, categorising, naming and labelling and putting into boxes and never finding out who we truly are, or why we are here.

Some of us are drawn to the ocean, some are drawn to the woods, some are drawn to horses or dogs; each person can find out what other species, ecosystems, pieces of land make them feel whole, make them feel like they are singing their own song. It is a life long journey which may mean that we move on and journey in different places, with different kin at different times; or we may find that we are quiet phlegmatic people who are happy and content to work away calmly in a particular place with a small group for many years. The important thing is to take up our own thread and follow it authentically.

Organisation in the body; the body as a community

Each individual cell is a very small ecosystem. The cells then work together to form the tissues and organs of our bodies, so our bodies can be viewed as a community of cells working together, or as several smaller communities of cells that form a larger ecosystem; interdependent specialised microcosms within a macrocosm. A further echo of this is seen with the individual organism within its community or ecosystem, fitting into larger macrocosms with the scale growing larger as we move from a local region up to the Earth, to the Universe.

Apart from the ecosystem formed by our own cells, we have bacteria and other micro-organisms living on our skin, up our noses, in our mouths, in the gastrointestinal tract and so forth; we actually have a cloud of them around us, an aura of microflora. The microflora works in harmony as part of our immune system when everything is in balance. However, if we do not have enough exposure to 'dirt', the community goes out of balance. If our soil/terrain becomes imbalanced due to stresses such as exposure to toxins, inappropriate nutrition, emotional stress, over expenditure of energy the ecosystem members may also become disrupted in their attempt to achieve a new balance. We are ecosystems that work well when there is dynamic equilibrium; we are always in motion, and hopefully the body is continually shifting and changing in response to its environment, making physiological adaptations which are the material expression of what is happening in spirit. Furthermore, as well as being ecosystems, we are habitats for all the microflora. We are a microhabitat within the larger community.

All ecosystems are organised, although this might not always be apparent to the un-tuned eye. However, it is important to realise that this is a dynamic organisational state with constant flux and change, shifting and balancing. Within each system the different elements depend on one another to carry out various functions and actions; the same is true of the cells, tissues and systems of our bodies.

Even the molecules that make up all the material world, whether living or inorganic or mineral will organise themselves; molecular self-organisation. A thing becomes more than the sum of its parts. Cells organise themselves too. They exchange information in various ways; it is the meaning that is conveyed by electromagnetic, chemical, vibrational or other means that is important. Interestingly, if two heart cells are separated from each other and placed in a petri dish of nutrients, they will stop pulsing regularly and start to fibrillate, display chaotic beating. However, if the two are placed together they will entrain, they will start to pulse in harmony, in a healthy rhythm pattern. Cells entrain other cells; tissues can entrain other tissues. Entrainment occurs within organisms and between organisms; there is a story about twin girls who were placed in separate incubators when they were born, according to hospital protocols. However, one thrived whilst the other did not. A nurse decided to break with the protocol and place the two girls together since they had been that way in the womb. Immediately, the healthy one put her arm around her sister and the sister's pulse and breathing normalised and became healthy, she became healthy and flourished. When we are separated out, we lose this effect; when we are connected by entrainment, there is a synergistic effect, a building of energy; the 'sum of the parts' effect. The concept of a self-organised system applies to cultures and societies as well as organisms or ecosystems.

Nineteenth-century physiology has been the dominant approach to the functioning of the human organism for over 100 years and is therefore deeply embedded in our epistemology; the approach is that of looking at surfaces, of generalising from information that has often been garnered from individuals who are living in unnatural surroundings; much of it is based on surface assumptions, much of it is based on the assumption that the body is merely a machine. For example, according to nineteenth-century physiology, we do not make more stem cells to repair and replace tissues such as those in the brain. It was assumed for a long time that once the brain is fully developed there is a gradual attrition of the cells, reducing function and cognition. However, it has been shown that in a natural environment the body will produce new stem cells that will migrate to the hippocampus (neurogenesis), and to other regions of the body to effect repairs. Stress and screen time can shut down this process. Believing the dictates of nineteenth-century reductionist, analytical physiology and anatomy also shuts down the potential for some of the more miraculous possibilities of allowing the body to carry out its natural functions as a self-healing organism, of seeing that our bodies are always perfect; that disease is precisely that—a lack of ease, a signalling that we need to pay attention so that we can see what shifts we need to make in our internal and external environment to move back to ease.

Tissues are the next level of organisation recognised in the body and are classified into four types—nervous, muscle, connective, epithelial.

Nervous tissue is excitable and carries electrical and chemical information around the body, stores it in the brains, and transmits information gathered from the internal and external environments to the brain to allow adaptations to occur; it carries impulses back to the organs to allow these adaptations to be carried out.

Connective tissue connects parts of the body together; the most fluid connective tissue is the blood, which essentially connects all our cells together. There are the cartilaginous tissues that are primarily concerned with stabilisation and maintaining shape; cartilaginous tissue includes the fasciae that connect our body together and which can store large amounts of residual emotional and physical stress or trauma. The bones are also connective tissue providing a rigid framework to allow us to move the way we do and are also traditionally seen as connecting us to our ancestors, holding their wisdom so that no knowledge is ever truly lost. If we have the patience to sit and listen to the wisdom of the Earth, to truly listen to our teachers, the plants and our other kin, then we can reach into our bones and reclaim the knowledge and wisdom of our ancestors. We can also reach in and discover the true story of their wounds and so start the deep work of healing the ancestors.

Muscle tissue does the work of movement. And has the ability to contract and relax to accomplish this work.

Endothelial tissue lines and covers the surfaces—it is protective, renews itself regularly and helps in the task of taking in information from our external environment; all endothelial tissue is from the same embryological origin, and therefore a stimulus applied in one area can effect change in more deeply seated endothelial linings—that is why taking a mucilage rich demulcent herb orally can soothe the lining of the bronchi or the bladder. Looking at our embryological development in the womb gives us further insights into our evolutionary path—one worth exploring for yourself. In the womb, we go through the whole evolutionary development, from the plant, through all the quintessential originals.

Tissues are organised into organs: organs are communities of tissues developed to do specialised work to support particular aspects of the work need to maintain the whole organism.

Orthodox anatomy and physiology organise the organs into systems: nervous, cardiovascular, respiratory, gastrointestinal, genito-urinary, muscular, skeletal, immune, endocrine, reproductive, integumentary or skin. These systems are artificial constructs; they are valuable at the beginning of studying the human form, but most parts of the body insist on belonging to more than one system and just won't adhere to those strict rules, narrow labels and restrictive boxes.

So, we see that on the physical level the body is made up of communities that hopefully co-exist, co-operate, communicate and support one another.

The same is true mentally as we have several brains within our body; the head-brain is thought by some to be made up of three brains, namely the reptilian brain or brainstem, the limbic system or emotional brain and the neocortex or analytical, conscious brain. We also have the heart-brain and the gut-brain and the sacral plexus which relates to our reproductive parts; quite possibly there are others that we have not yet turned our attention to.

Emotionally, we are also multi-faceted beings. You may have noticed that your behaviour is quite different with different people. This is because we have more than one aspect to our personalities and we choose (or don't) on some level which one will interact with a person, group of people or other scenario. These personalities include the different ages that we have experienced, our masculine and feminine sides, our inner parent, our adult, our elder, our inner teacher and may include many others. These different parts of our emotional self are our emotional community. As we have begun to see, it important for communities to be able to discuss or parlay and reach an agreement by consensus; otherwise, a riot may ensue.

It stands to reason that if we have several physical, emotional and mental communities within us then this must be true on a spiritual level too.

All these interior communities interact with the exterior communities to which we belong or with whom we interact from day to day.

Communication

In order for there to be healthy functioning within a community or ecosystem, there need to be connections and communications between the different parts; it is also true within a human being. We tend to think of the nervous system and endocrine systems as the communication systems in our bodies, although it is now becoming apparent that the old concept of the neuroendocrine system is more accurate than separating these two out. Other communication systems in the body include the blood circulation, the myofascial system, the interstitium and the energy channels.

We communicate with other members of our ecosystem community through pheromones, electromagnetic radiation, talking, touch and so on. All species communicate with each other; we all exchange information by these methods. Plants send pheromones into the air and send information through the mycorrhizal network within the soil (where this has not been damaged by clear felling of the forest, deep ploughing techniques and other actions which disrupt or destroy it). They also send electromagnetic information.

In order for communication throughout an ecosystem to happen there need to be highways so that the information can travel. Thus, the hedgerows have acted as a last forest for plants and animals in Ireland, but they have been decimated in recent times.

Think about the same issues within the body and within our society ...

Communication is a conversation. So, if you wish, you can choose to spend each day in dialogue with your internal and external environment. If you are cooking, it can be a conversation with the ingredients you are working with; if you draw, write, garden, it can be a conversation bringing healing and health into the universal scenario. You are not doing to something; you are working with. We co-create with, put in our feelings and so do they, we dream together. We dream the world and the world dreams us ... It feels completely different as we stop doing to, imposing our will. Instead, we ask a bigger question—not how does it feel to me or how does it feel to them, but does this feel like we are co-creating the health of our planet and our community?

It is that simple and that is the hardest part: we are culturally encouraged into wanting complicated, difficult, glamorous, tricky. However, although it is simple, it is elegant and beautiful. And from that simple beginning, it can become very complex—a simple air on a tin whistle or a full orchestra playing a symphony. It is hard work at first as one is exercising new muscles, but they will become stronger and more flexible. Not only is one using new muscles, one is learning a new language—one of truth, honesty and integrity. One will find the mind is beginning to recognise the colonising, alien ideas that have been implanted through schooling and that these need to be weeded out. This part of the process can be extremely challenging for the ideas may be deeply rooted; they may have been presented as the ultimate truth and unshakeable.

Not only will you start to use a new language to express yourself, but you will also listen differently. When one works this way, one starts to honour those we are working with. We no longer try to rescue other people, we no longer become their victims, we no longer perpetrate power stealing in any form (sometimes power stealing can be cleverly disguised as helping, healing, caretaking and 'I want to be like you'). There is no place for sentimentality in this way of communicating, just truth, and honesty. The fluffy, flaky version will start to be exposed. It will be replaced by the wild version, the natural version. We find the wildness within starts to have a voice; we are no longer tamed or domesticated; we reclaim our indigenous soul. Civilisation is a glamorously dressed up form of human domestication, of enslavement to the mechanistic, reductionist mindset that keeps humans feeling separated from Nature, seeing themselves outside the web; the ultimate result of this is separation from the very self and total disempowerment. All the power becomes stolen by that Cartesian machine which seeks to take power from all for itself in one huge lie; there is no machine; there is just an epistemological error, a falsehood. And some of those practising this falsehood are the fundamentalist liberals and 'guru healers'.

Connection and communication in the body

Within ourselves, there are many ways in which the parts of the whole communicate. The neuroendocrine system is often thought of as the main communication throughout the body, and we will explore this later in the upper cauldron. The blood and lymph are both connective tissues which we will examine later when we explore the heart and lungs in the Middle Cauldron. For now, we are going to focus on the musculoskeletal system with its bones, joints, fasciae, ligaments, tendons and so forth.

The musculoskeletal system

When treating this system, we have an opportunity to be hands-on, to do some practical, experiential work with patients and give them exercises to do at home to work along internal medicine, salves to rub on, herbs to use in baths. Touch and movement are primary therapies that are included in all traditional medicine cultures, as is some form of myofascial unwinding.

The skeletal system is made up of bones and the associated connective tissues such as ligaments, tendons, the muscles, fascia and interstitium and the articulations or joints formed by these tissues. One of the most exciting things I learned from a friend of mine who is studying embryology is that when the bones are being formed in the body the templates are first laid down as cartilage and then these templates do what plant cells do: they use turgor, liquid pressure against the cell wall, to give the form and the basis of the skeleton. So, in the womb, as embryos, one of the first beings that we express is that of *plant*. The trees really are part of our ancestry, and we know it when we are growing in utero.

The spine is like the World Tree with the bony casing protecting the central nervous system. The spine offers protection to the spinal cord, the central communication strand and the peripheral nerves branch out from it reaching the muscles, the skin and the organs, so each of the peripheral nerves has a correspondence to particular organs and their energy too. The vertebrae of the spine are designed to allow flexibility and movement but also to protect. At the lower end, the cauda equina of the nervous system (horse's tail) analogous to the roots into the lower world, connecting us to the Earth, emerges from the lower end of the spinal column from the sacrum.

The pelvic cage or basin encases and protects the elements of the Lower Cauldron, namely the digestive system, urinary organs and reproductive organs, and these are all connected to our nourishment and survival as individuals and also as a species. It is open at the base to allow birthing and also the elimination of waste.

In the thorax, the rib cage protects the Middle Cauldron (the heart and lungs, our liver, our solar plexus) and relates to our emotional wellbeing and connection and exchange.

At the top, the nervous system branches out into the brain and reaches up to the sky, protected by the skull and this relates to the Upper Cauldron. The skull provides protection for the brain and is made up of several bones joined by sutures. At birth, the sutures at the top of the skull are still open and take some time to fuse, so we are still open. Once the sutures are joined there is still some flexibility in them; minor subluxations or fixations can occur.

Along each side of the spine run long muscles that help the spine to do its work and to enhance the flexibility of our backbone.

Muscles and bones work together to give flexibility, strength and movement when they are in health. Physical, emotional, mental, spiritual trauma can cause them to lock up, to tighten and armour areas of the body; muscles and fasciae can immobilise joints. The fascial system also has an intimate relationship with the muscles and bones and can also hold tension patterns. The interstitium was formerly thought to be merely packing material but is now understood to be more like a shock absorber layer; it is a little like bubble wrap with little pocket 'airbags'. Trauma can cause some of these to become deflated or over-inflated which leads to problems.

Rocks give structure to the Earth; they can be seen as analogous to the skeleton and both act as reservoirs of mineral deposits. There is an exchange in and out of the bones, and they are not dead or static—they are living material—but the information moves more slowly than it does in other tissues. The rocks similarly do not move quickly or give up their information in a hurry; one has to slow down enough to sit with the stones. However, the rocks hold a particular memory of the land, it's ancestry, its history, the long-term memory, whilst the soil could be said to be part of the short-term memory an analogous to the skin. Energetically, our bones hold the wisdom and knowledge of our ancestors; none of it has been lost we just need to be willing to reach into them, to listen to them and to take time to hear what they will offer us. In many cultures the ancestors are seen as still present with us rather than removed to heaven above the sky or the depths of hell; they are talked to, and their counsel is sought; it is understood that their wisdom and experience is still with us today. What about our relationship with our ancestors? As we heal this relationship in ourselves the healing and support of the ancestors can start to flow through, we heal that connection and communication.

It is interesting to note that our kidney Chi, base Chakra or Lower Cauldron energy is considered to be composed of before-heaven or ancestral Chi and after-heaven Chi (what nourishment we gather in this lifetime). Healthy kidneys are essential for the conversion of vitamin D to the form we use to strengthen our bones, and for other aspects of bone health. Several people I have spoken to (and it is my own experience) believe that ancestral wounding can be held in the kidney/adrenal complex; when we work to clear this, much more energy is available, the flow from the ancestors, their support can come through again and replenish our vital force. We need to accept that the shadow side of our culture exists; enlightenment is not just about looking towards the light, it is also about bringing the shadow into the light, looking at it, processing it and working with it to bring it to health. Also, we may look to the wounds of our Mother, the Earth, and rush off to rescue her, but we need to remember that we are part of the Earth too. The best place to start caretaking and healing is within our own skins. We take responsibility for our own wounds, our own psychic hygiene.

The tectonic plates are in some ways analogous to the myofascial system. They can become twisted and displaced due to physical, emotional and spiritual trauma and when this happens to the tectonic plates it can result in earthquake, or earth tremor and volcanic eruption. Myofascial twisting from an emotional, mental or physical trauma that occurs in one part of the body can give symptoms in a far-removed region. This can be demonstrated by twisting the top of say the little finger and tracing this through to see how this can cause sensations in a region as far removed as the big toe of the opposite foot. In craniosacral therapy and similar healing modalities, the way that this is dealt with is myofascial release; one sits with the tissues, providing a safe space for the body to re-align itself, to unwind. It might mean that there is a degree of tremoring, of shifting, but the body moves back to a healthier alignment. This trembling or shaking or jerking is often seen when re-alignments are taking place; the body may shake, tremble, writhe or unwind. If there are deep scars or wounds, then these may mean that the body finds a compensation point. This means that if stress is felt the symptoms may play up again and this is a signpost for stress telling us to notice what our tissues, our gut-brain, our RAS are trying to alert us to so that we can make ourselves safe and healthy.

There are several types of connective tissue in the musculoskeletal system:

Ligaments bind bone to bone; the strong ties that connect the ancestral memories together. Ancestral memory includes race memory, cultural memory, clan memory, community memory, family memory, and connect to land memory, Earth memory, Universal memory.

Tendons connect the muscles to the lever system of the bones and articulations so that the skeletal muscles can do the work of moving the levers and making us mobile. The tendons include golgi receptors which allow the fast action reflex movements away from danger such as overstretching or heat or sharp objects. Tendons also allow for the slower conscious, deliberate movements of our body to occur. The bones give us the structure to allow movement, and our ancestral memory informs our ability to move and evolve as a society.

Cartilage provides lining and protection, strengthening joints and structures.

The myofascium also contains a lot of golgi receptors and is a far more active tissue than previously thought. It is highly involved in proprioception, nocioception and the visceral fasciae play a large role in interoception. It is probably that the interstitium also plays a big role in feelings of pain and held trauma since it acts like a shock absorber and can become scarred, inflamed or atrophied in response to trauma.

Plants have a different way of expressing their structure. They have cell walls, and the perennials have lignin and bark and cambium. Trees have the memory of the rings and the bark. Perhaps cell walls are analogous to cartilage. Perhaps bark and lignified structures are like bones?

The tension in the musculoskeletal system often accompanies great emotional or mental tension. In conditions such as fibromyalgia, a person has often tightened up after a physical trauma, infection or a period of intense emotional stress. Whiplash injuries can have a similar pattern. Even with arthritis, there is often a great deal of mental or emotional tension accompanying the pain and tightness in the joints. Is it possible that a rigid mind gives a rigid body and vice versa? How often do people who have a lot of stress clench their hands, shoulders or teeth during their sleep when we ought to be relaxed? If movement frees up the body will this help to free the mental and emotional aspects of ourselves to break out of the tension, or out of looping thought patterns, or thought patterns that no longer serve, or even to release old emotional traumas? People who take up yoga, tai chi, other stretching and flexing exercises often report that such things happen. The region of pain and stiffness can sometimes give insight into what is happening for the person. We need to learn not to be too rigid but rather to have a balance between tradition and flexibility to evolve. Traditionally, older generations and younger generations would relate and share together; this allowed the older generations to pass on their experience, their stories, to keep their memories alive and retain more fluidity rather than feeling redundant or becoming obsolete or easy targets. Older generations can actually be more flexible in their worldview because of wider life experience if not cornered into fear.

Some exercises for the musculoskeletal system

Distraction

The easiest way to describe this is: one places one's fingertips firmly (just firmly, not harshly) on the skin. Make sure that the fingers are relaxed and slightly spread in the relax posture so that they can sense into the tissues underneath their contact, and then move them in a circular or linear brushing/scrubbing action, slowly and gently. The movement encourages the skin and underlying fascia to loosen any tensions between them and the deeper tissues. It is done gently and methodically for about 10 minutes. The fingers are then gently lifted off the skin. Cream or oil can be applied before doing this so that the constituents thereof facilitate relaxation and help to break up deposits.

Sotai

Sotai is a Japanese technique. This is a simple version of the technique. For any restricted range of movement (for example rotation of the head, elevation of the shoulders, abduction of the leg). Get the person to perform the movement on each side of the body (left and right); observe which is more restricted and ask them which is more uncomfortable. Then get them to breathe in and then as they breath out to perform the movement on the easier side of the body. Repeat this 3–5 times, reminding them to breathe with the movement. Then get them to repeat this on the other side. Encourage them to repeat this several times during the day.

Body mirroring

We learn how to move by watching how others do it when we are small, at least in part. This means that we may inherit some of our posture and movement patterns. However, we know that it is possible to retrain our learned behaviours and this technique can help. Stand facing the person you are working with. You may find their posture is different depending on whether they are standing on a soft natural surface such as sand or earth rather than on concrete. Observe their posture—are they holding their head centrally or to one side, are they thrusting their chin forward or retracting their neck back? Are their shoulders at an even height, is one shoulder further forward than the other? Is their spine in a natural S curve or are any of the curves exaggerated or absent? How about their hips, are they even? Are their knees equally soft? Is one foot further forward than the other? Are their arms loose and relaxed? Are they clenching their hands? Most of us are not completely symmetrical but notice any tension or guarding patterns. Then explain you are acting as a mirror, copying their posture and do this, maybe exaggerate it a little. Then gradually talk them through as you move to a more relaxed, natural, healthy posture with all of the body in a toned, relaxed alignment. Use reassuring language (do not criticise) and encourage them to use their breath as they re-align. Most often people will comment on how they feel more relaxed, that it takes less energy to stand in alignment. And do take into account any accommodations they are making. Encourage them to practise this in front of the mirror for themselves at home to help them to habituate into a natural alignment.

Unwinding

We all do this naturally. Have you ever noticed yourself making little twitches or jerks as you are falling asleep; this is the body naturally unwinding from the tensions of the day. Sometimes it can be helpful to have someone hold a space for our bodies to relax into this, releasing physical or emotional tensions from the body. The process can be accompanied by yawning, stretching, belching, farting, a few tears, giggles or a bit of a rant as we let go. It is possible for several people to work on a person at the same time and often the being's inner healer will recognise who will be best at unwinding a particular piece in this situation. However, here is a description of one person working with one person.

Get the person who wishes to unwind to lie on a treatment couch. Make sure that they are comfortable and warm. Make sure that the couch is at a good height to ensure one's own posture is relaxed. Sitting on a pilates ball or a chair with casters is best so that one can move around the couch with ease. Start off by lightly making contact with the ankles, gently cupping them in your hands and focus into the person to access where to start working; one may receive this as a visual impression or an intuition. One may stay at the feet, feel drawn to holding the head, the abdomen or shoulders. Place the hands symmetrically, either laterally or over and under the body. The pressure one uses is that of a piece of paper or small coin; in other words, one does not use pressure. Become aware of any movements occurring—pulsing, micro flexions and so on in the musculature or fasciae. Listen with the fingers, sometimes it feels like what one does with a stuck drawer in an old dresser, just wiggling and easing until it loosens out rather than trying to pull and tug against the resistance. Tissues love to be eased and coaxed and encouraged, well don't we all prefer that to pulling and tugging? Follow these movements gently with your hands. If the arms or legs are being worked on, encourage the person to allow the limb to relax completely, give you the weight of it and then just wait to see if it moves. If it does then follow through the movements, just follow, do not lead. Then do the same if one is working on the neck. Sometimes the movements will go through a repeating arc, a loop of stuck patterning. If this is the case, one can either just hold the part being worked on static for a few seconds to see if that shifts it. Or one can just move slightly sideways to break the loop and allow release. It is important to realise that one is holding and following rather than directing; one is holding space and going with the flow rather than doing work to. Sometimes, the person will feel like huge movements are being made when it is just little micro stretches; sometimes one might find oneself mirroring their neck movements or yawning and stretching the jaw. It is also possible to do this work for one's self with a little practice.

Examples of herbs for the musculoskeletal system

Acanthus mollis, Achillea millefolium, Ananas comosus, Apium graveolens, Arctium lappa, Arnica montana, Bellis perennis, Betula species, Boswellia carterii, Brassica species, Calendula officinalis, Capsicum minimum, Centella asiatica, Cinnamomum verum, Curcuma longa, Echinacea angustifolia radix, Eleuthrococcus senticosus, Eucalyptus species, Eugenia caryophyllum, Filipendula ulmaria, Guaiacum species, Harpagophytum procumbens, Hypericum perforatum, Juniperus communis, Melaleuca species, Mentha species, Origanum vulgare, Plantago species, Qercus robur, Rumex crispus, Salix species, Symphytum officinale, Taraxacum officinale radix, Urtica dioica folia, Valeriana officinalis, Viburnum opulus, Withania somniferum, Zingiber officinale, Seaweeds.

Anti-inflammatories

Betula species, Salix alba, Filipendula ulmaria, Origanum vulgare, Cinnamomum verum, Achillea millefolium, Curcuma longa, Guaiacum officinale, Prunella vulgaris, Urtica dioica.

Sea salt and Epsom salt baths, cider vinegar internally and externally. Many types of poultices such as potato and mustard, cabbage, linseed.

Depuratives

Arctium lappa, Rumex cripus, Taraxacum officinale, Urtica dioica.

Antispasmodics

Mentha x piperita, Thymus vulgaris, Rosmarinus officinalis, Origanum vulgare, Valeriana officinalis, Matricaria recutita, Viburnum opulus, Salvia sclarea, Lavandula vera.

Circulatory stimulants

Capsicum minimum, Brassica species, Amoracia rusticana, Eucalyptus species, Rosmarinus officinalis, Achillea millefolium.

Pain relief

Passiflora incarnata, Valeriana officinalis, Filipendula ulmaria, Meleuca alternifolia, Eugenia caryophyllum, Hypericum perforatum, Mentha x piperita, Lactuca virosa, Matricaria recutita, Rosmarinus officinalis, Viburnum opulus, Citrus aurantium flos, Zingiber officinale, Lavandula vera, Ananas comosus, Guaiacum officinale.

Connective tissue repair

Echinacea angustifolia, Eleuthrococcus senticosus, Plantago species, Symphytum officinale, Withania somniferum.
Seaweeds, mushrooms, adaptogens.

Boundaries, an example

Our skin is our largest organ; it is a boundary between our inner and outer realities.

It picks up information from the external environment so that we can balance our inner environment to our external. Information from the skin, the metabolites it makes and the substances it absorbs are also carried to other parts of the body via the blood. For example, the vitamin D synthesised in our skin in response to ultraviolet radiation is carried first to the liver for the next stage of its formation and then to the kidneys where it is transformed into the form that plays a part in maintaining bone strength and our immune system.

The skin is not an inert barrier; it absorbs, manufactures, protects, excretes and sends information into our external environment via those secretions. Walking barefoot on the soil or working the soil with bare hands transmits that information into our environment; this gives information to the soil and to the plants about us, and they then adapt their physiology to ours to promote health, so we cause changes in our bioregion by walking barefoot, handling the soil and the plants, and exchanging our excrement with the soil. The skin prefers an acid environment pH of 5.5–6. A lot of plants like soil of that pH too.

The skin is from the same embryological epithelial tissue as the lining of the gut (which is why gut dysbiosis or irritation can show up as a skin condition). Both the skin and the guts have microflora. The Microflora or commensiles of the acid mantle of the skin and those that live in the gastrointestinal tract help to communicate with the external world and act as part of our immune system, helping to maintain appropriate boundaries as we explored with the immune system; those in the skin prefer a slightly acid environment, and sweating and saunas help to maintain a healthy population. Epithelium also forms the linings of other organs (which is why gut dysbiosis can contribute to irritable bladder, rhinitis, asthma and other conditions). The epithelium is designed to have an outer layer of dead cells that are continually sloughed off and replaced by new cells and therefore is a part of excretion into the environment, transmitting information about our physiological state into our ecosystem. This continual replacement is part of our protection too. This is similar to the leaf fall that occurs seasonally in deciduous trees and in evergreen plants in a less marked cycle (returning waste and information and food into the soil; shedding of unwanted material, it is an active metabolic process cycling information and nutrients, rather than a littering of excrement and unwanted waste).

The skin microflora, or integumentary microbiota

Our skin is covered by millions of friendly bacteria that create a healthy defence to pathogens once they are allowed to flourish and are not continually stripped or otherwise compromised. There may be 180 different species living on our skin. There is a specialised species that lives on the cornea of our eye that can cope with the high levels of salt and enzymes in our tears; there are also tiny mites that live in the follicles of our eyelashes.

By covering the skin and occupying the space, the friendly bacteria (there are a few fungi and protists too) fill an ecological niche and thereby prevent pathogens from getting a foothold. As with the guts, some species that have the potential to become pathogens live peaceably in the community, once the soil is healthy and the community of microflora is flourishing. For example, Staphylococcus aureus is present in the skin population of nearly half of people but causes no problems; health carers are more likely to carry it in their microflora. It will move into wounds and may also cause impetigo if the immune system is down. Staphylococcus epidermidis is closely related to S. aureus and produces bacteriocins, proteins used to kill off closely related bacteria. Some bacteria such as the dermabacter and brevibacteria prefer moist dark niches and produce strong odours as part of the protection they offer. The commensile bacteria of the microflora differ from pathogens in that they do not produce coagulase, an enzyme produced by invasive species to break through the cell wall into our cells.

Obviously, the healthier our diet and the better nourished our skin then healthier the commensal population. Sweating has been shown to balance the dermal microbiota; we need to sweat regularly; sebum secretions are probably also important. However, it is likely that they also respond well to strokes, being talked to, and contact with Nature.

We can glean a lot of information about someone from their skin, both by looking and by feeling. When conversing with a patient, there are many things we can take note of:

- Pigmentation, skin tone and texture.
- Pores for the secretion of sweat (our smell) and sebum (also part of our smell); our odour is affected by our colouring, our gender, our mood, our diet and other factors that determine our internal environment.
- Fat deposits; subcutaneous fat. Fat is an insulator; specifically, it reduces electromagnetic conduction. Fat is not inert; it is metabolically active and more permeable to certain fat-soluble forms of chemical information. It stores certain chemicals, including some hormones, and can act as a reservoir for toxins. Some of the fatty tissues in our bodies will produce oestrogen.
- Response of pain and stroking receptors; people need strokes for the reticular activating system to function well. If they do not get strokes but only experience pain, then the RAS will start to respond to this with a pleasure response.
- Temperature and response to heat and cold.
- A myofascial layer which is supposed to remind us of who we are, what shape we are. Trauma can get stuck in it and then we remember whom we are in that trauma rather than letting it pass through. Scars in the skin can be indicative of traumas.
- Also, look at the hair; the health of the hair can tell us a lot about our health. Although it is only the root of the hair that is alive, we can look at its strength, lustre, secretions of the scalp. Some people use hair analysis to detect deficiencies in the body. Hairdressers will tell you that the scalp secretions of people with conditions such as schizophrenia and depression are significantly different from others.
- Nails: white flecks can be due to hard manual work and knocks to the nail bed, or mineral deficiency. Easily splitting nails can be due to chewing, essential fatty acid or mineral deficiency. Pitted nails may be a form of psoriasis. Bow's lines are horizontal lines that denote a time of extreme physical or emotional stress/depletion. The colouration of the skin under the nails can help to indicate iron deficiency or cyanosis (oxygen depletion in the system). Splinter haemorrhages indicate heart or respiratory disease or knocks from hard physical work.

Could it be that our skin is a sensory brain, an aspect of our neurological system facilitating our sensory acuity and our reading of the heart of the world, the *Anima Mundi*, the constant stream of information that floods around us?

We could link it in with our brains as follows:

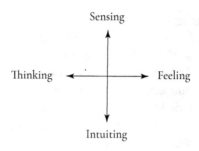

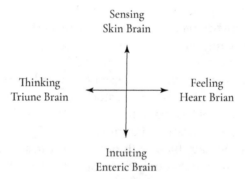

Fairly recently the skin was thought by scientists to be an impermeable barrier that prevented the absorption of active compounds into the body, yet it had always been used in traditional herbal medicine in delivery systems such as plasters, foot baths, sitz baths ointments and so forth. Nowadays the transdermal route is used for the delivery of a number of pharmaceutical medicines validating the traditional applications. The skin is the largest organ in the body, with a surface of approximately 1.8 metres square, which is a vast area of application. The skin is not inert; it is involved in respiration, absorption and elimination. However, whilst elimination and respiration are active processes, requiring work, absorption often occurs by simple diffusion.

The outer keratinised layer or *stratum corneum* (horny layer) is partly lipophilic and partly hydrophilic, meaning that it is partially permeable to both water-soluble and fat-soluble molecules. Since essential oils contain small molecular weight molecules of both types, they tend to permeate the skin quite readily, but molecules over 500 molecular weight hardly penetrate at all.

What factors affect the number of active constituents of herbs and oils actually absorbed into the bloodstream?

- The surface area of application. Obviously, the larger the area of application, the more is absorbed. However, if areas are left uncovered, then most of the volatile components will evaporate, rather than passing through the skin.
- The permeability of skin on different regions of the body; the most permeable regions are the soles of the feet, the palms of the hands, the forehead, armpits, damaged, abraded or inflamed skin, mucous membranes, the scalp. The least permeable areas are the buttocks, abdomen, trunk and legs.
- The viscosity of any carrier used. The more viscous oils such as almond and olive oil permeate more slowly, whereas a low viscosity oil, such as linseed, permeates more quickly. The fatty acid composition of the carrier oil will also affect the rate of absorption.
- Hydration of the skin: skin that is waterlogged from immersion in hot water. Although the *stratum corneum* on the soles and the palms are many times thicker than on other parts of the body, it has a tendency to take up water. So, the traditional foot bath is an excellent system of delivery. If the skin has been previously washed with detergents, it will be even more permeable.
- The temperature of the oil/compress/poultice/bath, the client's skin and the environment will all affect the rate of absorption. About 10°C is sufficient to increase absorption several fold, and the circulatory stimulating effect of massage will no doubt enhance this.
- Occlusion, or covering the skin with non-permeable material will also have an effect. This does not mean that you should wrap your clients in cling film. Merely covering areas where application has taken place with towels, and the client dressing in normal outdoor clothes after a treatment should suffice. Recently the possibility of skin enzymes breaking down certain molecules has also been investigated as a factor that affects the dosage.
- Greasy ointments, especially those containing lanolin or mineral oils, will hinder absorption and are not suitable media for application.

However, vegetable oil-based lotions and cream increase the permeability of the skin and therefore are useful media, especially for the patient to use between treatments.

Examples of herbs for the skin

Achillea millefolium, Allium sativum, Althea species, Arctium lappa, Avena sativa, Bellis perennis, Berberis aquifolium et vulgaris, Calendula officinalis, Centella asiatica, Chicorium intybus, Cxitrus aurantium flos, Crateagus species, Curcuma longa, Glycyrrhiza glabra, Hamamelis virginiana, Hypericum perforatum, Lavandula species, Linum usitatissimum, Matricaria recutita, Melaleuca alternifolia, Origanum vulgare, Pelargonium species, Plantago species, Pogostemon cablin, Rosa species, Rosmarinus officinalis, Rumex crispus, Scrophularia nodosa, Stellaria media, Symphytum officinale, Taraxacum officinale, Theobroma cacao, Tilia species, Trifolium pratense, Urtica dioica, Vetiveria zizanoides, Viola tricolor.

Alteratives and depuratives

Arctium lappa, Berberis species, Chicorium intybus, Curcuma longa, Glycyrrhiza glabra, Rumex crispus, Taraxacum officinale, Urtica dioica.

Antiallergic, itching skin

Althea officinalis, Calendula officinalis, Citrus aurantium flos, Curcuma longa, Glycyrrhiza glabra, Hamamelis virginina, Lavandula species, Matricaria recutita, Plantago species, Stellaria media, Tilia species, Trifolium pratense, Viola tricolor.

Lymphatics

Calendula officinalis, Echinacea angustifolia, Scrophularia nodosa, Trifolium pratense, Viola species.

Diaphoretics and herbs to improve circulation

Achillea millefolium, Mentha x piperita, Sambucus nigra flos, Tilia species, Crateagus specis, Vaccinium myrtillus.

Cicatriscants

Achillea millefolium, Calendula officinalis, Hypericum perforatum, Lavandula species, Rosa species, Rosmarinus officinalis.

Emollients/demulcents

Althea, Avena, Glycyrrhiza, Linum, Plantago, Symphytum, Theobroma, Tilia.
Also, a wide range of nut and seed oils and butters, aloe vera, seaweeds.

Bruises

Bellis, Hamamelis, Lavandula, Pelargonium ol., Plantago, Symphytum, Foeniculum ol., Origanum marjorana ol.

Bites and stings

Bellis, Helichrysum, Lavandula, Melaleuca, Plantago, Rumex fol.

Scars

Boswellia, Citrus aurantium, Helichrysum, Lavandula, Pogostemon, Rosa, Rosmarinus officinalis ct. verbenone, Vetiveria.

Skin ulcers and varicose eczema

Calendula officinalis, Zanthoxylum, Zingiber, Crataegus, Matricaria, Hamamelis, Melaleuca, Commiphora, Allium sativum.
Local wild honey.

Acne and bacterial infections

Echinacea angustifolia, Allium sativum, Commiphora molmol, Juniperus communis ol., Baptisia, Calendula officinalis, Inula.

Viral infections

Glycyrrhiza glabra, Mentha x piperita, Lavandula officinalis, Hypericum perforatum, Calendula officinalis, Melissa officinalis, Echinacea angustifolia rad., Eucalyptus.

Fungal infections

Azadirachta, Calendula, Cinnamomum ol., Origanum ol., Thymus vulgaris, Pelargonium graveolens, Eucalyptus sp., Matricaria recutita, Melaleuca species, Lavandula officinalis, Commiphora molmol ol.
      Also consider treating the liver, bowel, kidneys and lungs to optimise other routes of elimination.

The scars of trauma serve to remind us of the path that led us to become who we are today. The wounds heal as the lessons are learned, the scars (preferably just hairlines) stay lest we forget the lessons and need to be reminded of the pain of birthing ourselves (which we do over and over again).

A meditation with the skin of the earth: the soil

The soil is one of the most incredible ecosystems on the planet. It is not just an inert substrate for plants to stick their roots into. It breathes, it is full of all sorts of micro-organisms, it is alive. When the soil is deep-dug or deep ploughed it destroys the web of life within this ecosystem. In a teaspoon of soil there are thousands of strands of mycorrhizae (the filamentous threads that make up the bodies of fungi and that form intimate relationships with the roots of plants, either wrapping around them ecto mycorrhizae or penetrating into them endomycorrhizae), there are millions of micro-organisms such as bacteria, actinomycetes, yeasts, protozoa and algae and there are the ones visible to the naked eye such as earthworms, nematodes, mites, slugs and snails. There are different textures and types of soil depending on what it is mainly composed of and where it is. Soil contains loam, hummus, sand, minerals, clay and other particles.
      Soil is affected by rainfall, frost, drought and is fed by the plants living in it as they drop their leaves or decompose at the end of their lives; it is also fed by animal and bird excrement and the decomposition of creatures when they reach the end of their life. Nutrients in the soil are broken down by the vibrant life forms that live in it. These creatures help the soil to breathe and drain. Nitric acid in the atmosphere is brought down to earth by lightning. The healthier the soil is for all the micro-organisms, the healthier the plants that grow in it and therefore the better the food and medicine they provide. Some plants find it really

hard to grow without their symbiotic mycorrhizae; for example, roses. Soil organisms are damaged by high temperatures when the soil is left bare and tilled. A healthy soil ecosystem is encouraged by as little digging as possible, as little compaction as possible (walk lightly on the Earth), the right pH and organic mulch. It is a fascinating thing to sit with a patch of soil and really notice what is going on.

In the same way that we can sit with a plant to learn more of its story, we can also sit with a patch of soil. So, with your heart centred and your inner child accompanying you go outside and find a patch of soil to sit with. When you visit new places, take some time to sit with the soil. Even better, also take off your shoes and let your feet feel the soil, get your hands into the soil and feel it. Notice the texture, the colours, the smell. Does the soil feel healthy? Is it breathing? Does it need anything? So much of our soil has been deeply insulted by over digging, undernourishment (soil needs a wholesome diet of compost, manure and seaweed, rather than artificial fertilisers)? Has the soil been overworked or depleted by intensive cropping? Healthy soil has the most amazing smell, texture and colour. Soil that is well nourished is simply delicious to the senses, and no I haven't tried eating it, but sometimes it looks good enough.

Herbs for the whole human

All herbs are of benefit to the whole person and sometimes we just need to work with one. As we move through the body systems, we will look at many allies and listen to their stories. However, there are two specific actions that herbs have that can be of value for the whole system, and so we will introduce the concept of plant therapeutic actions or properties here in order to start weaving that thread into the tapestry.

We love putting things into boxes and categories. As part of the process of learning, this can be very valuable as it can help us to start to form a picture. With the actions of herbs, it is important to realise that, being complex medicines from whole plants, herbal medicines may well have many actions. Also, the action of a herb can depend on the form used, the therapist using it, the person taking it and the combination of herbs used. In some instances, the action of a herb is due to one major constituent, but in most cases the action is as a result of the synergy between the different constituents (the sum of the whole is greater than the parts of the whole); the different constituents may quench, buffer, potentise, increase bioavailability. Although we will take the chemistry of the plants into consideration, the main focus will be on the overall character and nature of the plant.

Adaptogens

These herbs help the body deal with stress; they work on strengthening and adapting our basic ability to deal with physiological, physical, mental, emotional and spiritual stressors. The person becomes more resilient to stress and external pressure so that we can deal with more of it before it impinges on our health. They definitely support the adrenal glands, may help with tissue repair, modulating the immune system and much more besides. It is important to realise that it is most beneficial to use them alongside good nutrition, proper hydration, appropriate exercise, meditation and other relaxation techniques.

Examples:

Angelica archangelica, Arctium lappa, Astragalus membranaceous, Bacopa monnieri, Centella asiatica, Eleutherococcus senticosus, Ganoderma lucidum, Glycyrrhiza glabra, Levisticum officinale, Ocimum sanctum, Panax ginseng, Rhodiola roseum, Rosmarinus officinalis, Schisandra chinensis, Scutellaria baiacalensis, Stachys betonica, Urtica dioica, Withania somniferum, Codonopsis membraneus, Inula helenium, Sambucus nigra fructus, Salvia officinalis, Thymus vulgaris, Rosa canina fructus, Vaccinium myrtillus fructus.

Alteratives

These herbs support a return to healthy function in the body. They work gradually to increase the health and vitality of a person. Some seem to have a general influence on the person whilst others support specific processes such as waste elimination via the lungs/liver/skin/kidneys or else stimulate specific systems such as digestive function and elimination or the immune system. This is one action that has not found its way into the language of modern biomedicine. Some of these herbs are clearly therapeutic medicines whilst others are on the borderline between food and medicine. Remember that in Galenic terms there are the four degrees of intensity of action: first degree is strong medicine/poison, second is strong medicine, third is gentle medicine and fourth is a food. Sometimes the differentiation is dose-dependent.

Examples:

Allium sativum, Anemone pulsatilla, Anthriscus cerefolium, Arctium lappa, Azadirachta indica, Baptisia tinctoria, Berberis aquifolium et vulgaris, Chionanthus virginicus, Cimicifuga racemosa, Echinacea angustifolia, Erythrea centaurea, Fumaria officinalis, Galium aperine, Gentiana lutea, Glycyrrhiza glabra, Hydrastis canadensis, Iris versicolor, Menyanthes trifoliata, Prunella vulgaris, Rumex crispus et acetosa et acetosella, Scrophularia nodosa, Smilax spp., Trifolium pratense, Urtica dioica, Viola odorata et tricolor.

Oak (daur) a tree of community

One of the greatest medicines that this tree provides is sitting under its shade. In pre-Christian times, oaks were planted to mark boundaries and large, solitary oaks were law trees, a place to meet to make judgements and decisions for the community; they were also places where wedding ceremonies were held.

Many years ago, Ireland and most of Europe was covered with oak forest, but we all know that this was removed to use in building dwellings and constructing ships that were used for waging war or colonising other regions of the world. Since oak is a climax species in forests, it had taken hundreds of years for the forests to evolve to this point with many other species acting as pioneers, such as birch trees which sweeten the soil, and wolves who help forestation by protecting the trees from grazing animals. Only small areas of primary forest remain. However, the oak is superbly suited to the Irish climate and will reach a great age if left to mature, or coppiced with proper carefulness; when coppiced with respect and attention to what the tree needs, its lifespan can be doubled or tripled. The planting of an oak forest by a community is a commitment to care for hundreds of years (an oak tree can live for about 1000 years) to teach the new generations how to listen to the trees, care for them and in turn receive the sacred protection and resources that the forest provides in return.

We tend to think of the mighty spreading oaks found in isolation in fields and parkland as examples of the older trees; however, in a forest, there may be oaks of great seniority that have not achieved such great girth due to the fact that they are growing within the community of the forest. An individual oak in isolation will grow big and tall to express sufficient oakness in a place surrounded by smaller allies such as grasses and meadow flowers and shrubs; where oaks grow close, there is enough oakness expressed by smaller, thinner individuals all saying we are oak together. Oak helps us to remember who we are and access the profound connection to a bigger community. The word 'robust' comes from the species name for one of our oaks, robur, and the oak can truly help us find our strength, our anchoring in the here and now, and find our authentic self within the community, the individual that supports and contributes and in turn is fed and supported. Oak helps us to remember who we are and access a profound connection to a bigger community. Anchored in the present, the community can dream the emergence of a beautiful future, and work to bring it into being.

CHAPTER EIGHT

The lower cauldron physical survival of the individual and species (reproduction)

The Lower Cauldron is known as the cauldron of Warmth or Incubation and is centred in our pelvis like the lower burner or Daitinen or Hara of Eastern Medicine philosophy. We are born with this cauldron upright, a bowl of vitality which gives us our physical, health, mobility and life force.

The Lower Cauldron needs to be full, relaxed and nourished in order for us to survive and thrive both as an individual and then as a species. When it is full, it provides heat and energy for our whole being and allows the Middle Cauldron to fill. Its original Celtic name was Coire Goirath.

So, in this section, we will look at the digestive system, including the liver and its connections to anger, determination and planning, the spleen and worry, the pancreas, solar plexus and the gut-brain. We will also explore the kidney-adrenal complex and its association with fear and courage. Then we will explore the sacral plexus and our reproductive organs and their connection with creativity.

The gastrointestinal system (GIT)

The gastrointestinal system is sometimes called our digestive system. However, this is something of a misnomer, since it does a lot more than that and also our essential nutrients are not all taken in or digested in the GIT and include:

- Oxygen (via the lungs but also acts on the skin)
- Water
- Food (carbohydrates, fats, protein, fibre, vitamins, minerals and wild food—see below for more about this component)
- Love
- Light (by the photoreceptive tissues in our eyes and other areas of the body)
- Connecting with Nature
- Sensory stimulation—sound, sight, smell, taste, touch, good electro-magnetic radiation and others

With each nutrient, too little or too much will lead to illness or death. For example, sunlight does not cause disease; we need it. However, if we spend most of our time without this nutrient and then gorge on it inappropriately then health problems will occur. In traditional cultures people adapt their time outside to be in step with light; the function of the siesta was in part to spend that time of day in the shade. Sunlight enables us to produce vitamin D in our skin; taking Beta carotene helps protect the skin against light damage, protects against UV radiation (or even better eat plenty of carotenoid-rich foods, including carrots, sweet peppers and wild greens); plants use carotenoids as photosynthetic molecules for harvesting light and also to protect against excess UV radiation. Also, flavonoids, particularly anthocyanins, are produced to protect plants against UV radiation, as are certain essential oil constituents and other molecules. Research is beginning to be carried out into the benefits of including plants that have adapted to protect themselves against excess radiation into the diet as a way of protecting ourselves.

The value of including wild or hunter-gather foods in the diet is also being investigated. These are sometimes referred to as famine foods since they would have supplemented the diet at lean times of the year. Our ancestors would have made use of a far wider range of foodstuffs than those we limit ourselves to these days; we have limited our food plants to around 30 out of a potential few hundred locally, and several thousand globally.

Research is beginning to suggest that eating wild foods can be of great benefit and this is borne out by looking at more traditional cultures and their health. People following such a diet are eating local food (exposed to the same environmental factors), which is in season. The food tends to be very fresh or preserved by more natural methods such as drying, fermenting or pickling. What is also emerging is the benefit of the micronutrients in these foods. These include chemicals that can be toxic in large amounts, but in small amounts stimulate the immune system into healthy function. The diet contains small amounts of a wider range of foods; one would graze on small amounts of what is in season getting a huge variety of information through the diet. Many of the substances in these plants have medicinal benefits, plenty of antioxidants, anti-inflammatories, different fibres that slow down simple sugar and saturated fat absorption, plant proteins, prebiotics that encourage a healthy gut flora, immuno-modulators and much more. It is also apparent that local game or domestic animals that have grazed on a wide range of foods and got plenty of exercise have a better fat profile in their meat, less saturated fats, more omega 3 fats; and they play an important role in the health of the ecosystem. It would appear that these more natural eating practices prevent the occurrence of many of the disease of Western society.

By following the foods in season, there can be many benefits, for example:

Tomatoes contain lycopene which protects against sunburn, and they ripen during the sunniest part of the year. Elderberries are produced at a time of year when our immune systems need a bit of a boost. Elderflowers are produced around the hay fever season. Nettles are a timely spring tonic along with other emerging greens such as chickweed, bittercress, dock leaves and ramsons. The staple root crops that traditionally nourish us through the winter are a valuable source of inulin, a polysaccharide which is hugely beneficial for our immune system, and our bones (at a time of lower vitamin D synthesis); the lists could go on forever. Researchers started to look at the implications of ingesting higher quantities of micronutrients in the diet in the early part of this century. They noted that primates, such as chimps, ingest huge quantities of plant food which meant a higher level of dietary intake of substances such as vitamin C, and other vitamins, also of specific minerals that are concentrated in a plant-rich diet. They concluded that the wild plant-based diet was serving important immunological and other beneficial functions.

Some examples

When following a traditional lifestyle, the Masai get about two-thirds of their daily calorie intake from milk and meat products and a third from wild forest plants. Additionally, their cattle are feeding on wild food rather than monoculture grass, or processed food. Many of the wild foods contain valuable micronutrients, including vitamins and minerals. When they follow this lifestyle, the Masai do not develop the same health problems displayed by Westerners eating a meat-rich diet. There could be several factors involved here; first, they supplement their diets with the forest foods; second, they are not sedentary; third, their animals are not factory reared; fourth, both the people and the animals are spending all their time in Nature; it is their home. As urbanisation occurs and they move from their traditional way of life they tend to start to develop more and more Western diseases.

A similar situation has been seen with middle-aged Asian men. The incidence of late-onset diabetes becomes greater as these people move towards Western diets and lifestyles. However, if they are given dietary and lifestyle counselling to remind them of their traditional ways, their symptoms disappear within six weeks without recourse to medication—the disease disappears.

The village of Acciaroli in Italy attracted interest from researchers in Rome's Sapienza University and the Sandiego School of Medicine due to the fact more than 1 in 10 of the population of 700 people is over 100 years old. The researchers found that the inhabitants of the region have excellent blood circulation in comparison to other people of their age, with low blood levels of adrenomedullin similar to people in their 20s or 30s. High levels can cause circulatory problems due to the contraction of blood vessels. It is believed this is down to their diet of fish, locally reared chickens and rabbits, homegrown fruit and vegetables and large amounts of rosemary. The people of the region do not have chronic disease associated with older people in other regions such as heart disease, Alzheimer's, cataracts or obesity. They stay physically active and well.

Grivetti and Ogle wrote a fascinating paper entitled *Value of traditional macro and micronutrient needs: the wild plant connections* in which they discuss how edible wild foods have been known to be valuable since antiquity; as medicinal plants have. They make the point that it is only recently that people have started to research them; also, a bit like medicinal plants. They point out there is little profit in such exercises and that such investigations are cross-disciplinary, and there has not been sufficient communications between the different faculties, that there is a lack of adequate conventional databases since much of the knowledge is shared by verbal communication which limits the educational efforts in using these plants to improve dietary health in developing regions. This highlights the problems that occur when the Western reductionist colonisers go in and destroy verbal lore, the traditional databases, and then throw our hands up. We do not put money into recovering the information for those we have stamped it out from; there is no product at the end of it so who would fund such a thing? In our own fields, some particularly delicious wild food plants are dismissed as weeds of agriculture; fat hen and the other chenopodiums are as good as, if not better than, spinach. These grow widely as 'weeds of agriculture' because they were once the crops raised by Neolithic peoples. Fat hen is our 'native quinoa' and was raised as both a leaf and a seed crop. The seeds of this plant and others such as nettle are full of most nourishing proteins, a great range of fatty acids vitamins and minerals; equal to, or surpassing, many of the imported superfoods.

On immunological and many other levels, we can consider how eating the wilderness brings us in touch with our local environment, bringing meanings into our bodies, feeding the meanings to our gut-brain so that we can make sense of where we are living and adjust our physiology accordingly. If we then return our physiological information into that environment (through the use of our excrement as manure, by walking barefoot on the earth, by working with the soil with our bare hands, by sucking seeds gently in our mouths before planting them) then it becomes a two way conversation with the plants adjusting to us and us likewise to them, an intriguing idea; truly reconnecting with the web. It is a conversation, not a technique.

Moving onto the gastrointestinal system, which is partly about digestion and absorption, but there's really a lot more going on, and a lot more connections to be made. Rather than the gastrointestinal system in isolation, we now need to consider the brain-enteric-gut-microbiota complex. There is a huge amount of new research in this area compared to what is in the conventional A&P texts. More recent research has shown that our concept of what the guts do is severely restricted—they have an important role to play in our endocrine, nervous and immuno-logical function, as well as digesting and absorbing and excreting on a physical level (and on other levels if we wish to take a more energetic approach). We also need to look into what relevance this has to how we understand our plant medicines and our food, and how we work with them.

In evolutionary terms, the enteric brain was the first to evolve. The first nerves evolved in the guts; it's a complicated business to co-ordinate digestion, making sure enzymes, acid and all the other right things are secreted in the required quantities and that the entire incredibly long length of the gastrointestinal tract moves, churns and squeezes at the rate that allows food to be adequately digested, the nutrients absorbed and the unneeded portions excreted. So, nerves were evolved to help coordinate all this activity. Then the reptilian part of the triune brain evolved, with the limbic system and neo-cortex getting added further along the way. In embryological terms the ENS and the CNS develop from the neural crest; this tissue divides as the embryo develops to form the two separate brains; as we know with tissues that have that embryonic connection, a close association continues into the fully developed human. The ENS is composed of about 100 million neurons and carries out autonomous function even if connections with the CNS are severed. However, the two brains are connected via both the sympa-thetic and parasympathetic branches of the autonomic nervous system, allowing information to flow in both directions between them. The ENS has support cells for the neurons and ganglia that make them up and a diffusion barrier similar to the blood-brain barrier to protect against infections and poisons. Both the triune brain and the ENS also have two layers; the mesenteric layer is found in the muscle layer of the gut wall and is involved in muscle function (peristalsis and so forth) and the submucosal plexus in the submucosa which is involved in controlling secretion. The ENS secretes and responds to neurotransmitters such as serotonin, acetylcholine, nitric oxide, dopamine and benzodiazepine-like substances; something like 95% of the body's serotonin is found in the gut. The serotonin produced in the gut cannot cross the blood-brain barrier, only 5HTP (which converts to serotonin) can. However, there is evidence to suggest that a happy gut-brain will help the head-brain to produce serotonin. The gastrointestinal tract also secretes hormones in the stomach, pancreas and small intestine; these help to control the functions of the digestive system, but many of them have also been shown to act as neurotransmitters and neuromodulators in the rest of the nervous system. The electromagnetic field of the enteric brain reads the information from foods and medicines and anything that we ingest in order to determine whether it is nourishing or toxic. Babies and children who put everything in their mouths are building up a library or database of information for the gut-brain and the immune system. The two layers or networks of the gut-brain use different neural pathways; the first analyses the electromagnetic information and uses dopamine as the main neurotransmitter, and the second needs to calibrate with taste and then uses electromagnetic information and its main neurotransmitter is serotonin.

Both the heart and the guts have a pacemaker. The gut pacemaker is the interstitial cells of Cajal which sends out rhythmic pulses in a similar way to the pacemaker in the heart. It is quite possible, indeed likely, that these two pacemakers can entrain and that heart coherence work can improve bowel function. The heart is a stronger neural and electromagnetic resonator, so it is more likely that the heart will entrain the gut; however, extremely strong signals from the gut may disrupt the heart energy—there are always feedback mechanisms in the body.

It has also been discovered that diseases that affect the CNS are echoed in the gut. The amyloid plaques formed in Alzheimer's are found in both the brain and the gut; the Levvy bodies of Parkinson's are also found in both locations.

When we experience stress, the ENS shuts down the digestive processes and initiates an inflammatory response. This allows energy to be temporarily diverted to running away or fighting; the inflammatory response prepares the immune system to heal any injury to the guts and to prevent infection in wounds. This system works well when stress is temporary; it works when stress is a short-term crisis that is dealt with and then a more parasympathetic/heart/cholinergic pattern would re-establish until the next emergency. Chronic, persistent stress means that digestion is continually delayed, and that the GIT is permanently inflamed which can lead to conditions such as Crohn's, colitis, IBS, indigestion, migraine, food intolerance, to weight gain, type II diabetes, hyperlipidaemia and other conditions associated with the digestive system. Since information flows in both directions, there can also be mental and emotional effects from constant physical gut irritation. If the gut lining is inflamed from exposure to antibiotics, heavy metals, foods that do not suit, then there can be detrimental effects on mood and outlook; the guts can initiate thoughts, behaviours and emotions. This means that problems in the gut or a stressed ENS can lead to depression, anxiety, panic attacks, ADD or ADHD. By treating the gut, the emotions and behaviours can move back towards balance.

The ENS can trigger the fear, flight and fight response. One simple test for food sensitivities or intolerances can be to test the pulse rate after eating—if it becomes elevated then this indicates a sensitivity to the food. Elevated pulse rate is part of the adrenal response. This has huge implications as regards the types of food that we eat and the information it gives us about our environment. Since we are by nature part of Nature if we only eat synthetic, highly processed food, then our guts will get alarmed. If we include local fresh and wild foods, then our ENS gets the message that we are at home in the place we need to be, connected into the web. Remember also that the buccal cavity is a highly enervated area and that eating is a tactile experience as well. This may also give us some insight into why some foods are inflammatory whilst others are anti-inflammatory; inflammatory foods give us messages that send us into the HPA fear, flight, fight response, and anti-inflammatory foods feed the parasympathetic; heart/cholinergic axis which involved with rest, repair, restore, relax, nurture and nourish.

The microbiota

The GIT is inhabited by 10^3–10^4 microbes; this is about ten times as many cells as there are human cells in our bodies. There are probably about 1000 species in there including bacteria (mostly anaerobes), viruses, protozoa, archaea and fungi. There may be a few worms too! Really it is very similar to a compost heap or a healthy soil ecosystem in its diversity. There are organisms living in the entire length of our GIT from the buccal cavity to the anus. The colonisation of the gut starts in infancy, and the initial microbiota will have a maternal signature for obvious reasons. The un-weaned child has a relatively simple gut flora, and it tends to be more individualised. The population size and diversity of this community increases with environmental exposure and with a widening diet so that by the time the child is 1-year-old the microbiome has become more complex and more similar to that of the adult. Environmental exposure to 'good dirt' is important for the development of the gut flora and also therefore the immune system. Fermented foods have been shown to help balance the gut flora. These were traditionally produced in each home or at least on a local level. Thus, the fermentation process and organisms were adapted to the same environment as those eating the fermented products thus adapting the gut flora to the local environment. Now, these products are often produced in large factories with everything being sterilised. Such products have been shown to be less beneficial as regards probiotic activity.

A diet high in processed foods, especially refined sugars and carbohydrates and food additives may well have a huge effect on the development of this population. Although there is huge individuality in the gut flora, there are certain population ranges that enhance health. Factors such as infection, disease, diet, stress and antibiotics can alter the gut flora, but it will tend to revert to its keynote stable diversity once the distorting factor has subsided.

We tend to hear about the fungal part of our gut flora only when it goes out of balance to become a 'pathogen' in the form of candidiasis. The candida organism is part of our healthy gut flora. However, when it forms an overgrowth, this can become a problem. But what if the candida only starts that overgrowth as an attempt to balance the environment in which it grows? Often, the overgrowth occurs in people who have large amounts of mercury in their systems from filllings (reduce heavy metals and it might drop?) or who have had large numbers of antibiotics killing off the bacteria (perhaps in this instance they are filling that niche left behind?), who are immune-compromised as a result of medication or disease—perhaps they are trying to supplement the intestinal immune function, or possibly to protect the lining of the gut from further damage, or to balance the pH. In addition, they will feed off high levels of certain substances if too much sugar or refined carbohydrate is taken in: they are trying to mop up the excess. A more holistic view would be to balance the environment to allow these valuable yeasts to reduce their population down to a sustainable level; if heavy metal toxicity is the trigger, use organisms such as chlorella, blue-green algae, spirulina, other seaweeds and medicinal mushrooms to remove these from the system; all algae and fungi which fill a similar niche in the larger ecosystem. Also, use medicine like *Rumex, Arctium, Coriandrum* to flush out the heavy metals. Bitters can help by stimulating the production of bile which is our natural gut flora balancer. Use seaweeds, and fibre rich foods such as stewed apple and herbs such as *Ulmus*, *Althea radix* as prebiotics to provide a good growing medium for healthy flora at the same time.

Worms are a really interesting one. Our culture tends to be revolted at the idea of having these 'parasites' as part of our intestinal fauna, but researchers found that a few of these guys can benefit our immune systems by reducing certain immune overreactions which cause atopic reactions (allergies) and autoimmune disease. Worms have been successfully used to treat conditions like Crohn's disease or even MS. The worms inhibit the action of Th17 cells and augment the activity of regulatory T cells which inhibit Th1, Th2 and Th17 cells; Th17 cells are particularly implicated in inflammatory diseases. If we go back 50 years or so, allergies were relatively uncommon in the Western world, and worms were still enjoying a relatively good relationship with humans. As worms were eradicated, allergies rose. In other parts of the world where worms are still relatively common the incidence of allergies is much lower. Also, people tend to live in a closer relationship with Nature in general—is it the worms or the relationship? Well, the fact that using worms to treat Crohn's works shows that it is part of the picture—it helps to redress that relationship.

Our gut flora are involved in our gut motility (the CNS, and ENS are also involved in this). The composition of our gut flora will affect how well we maintain the barrier function of the epithelium of the GIT. The healthier the gut flora, the higher the turnover of epithelial cells; because the epithelial cells in all our organs and in our skin are from the same embryonic origin, we start to see how important gut health is in treating any of the mucosa and our skin.

About 70% of our immune system is in our guts. There are cells in the small intestine that secrete a large variety of antimicrobial peptides, but they will only do this if the microflora is complete. The microflora are also essential for the development of the gut-associated-lymphoid tissue; this tissue is important as regards IgA secretion and controlled inflammation (a healthy immune response). Insufficient gut flora can lead to decreased plasma cells, decreased expression of activation mark-ers on intestinal macrophages, decreased nitric oxide levels, decreased histamine levels in the small intestine. There will also be less and smaller Peyer's patch follicles and mesenteric lymph nodes. But the good news is that re-colonisation will reverse this. Wildfood/herbs/hunter-gather foods in the diet may well be very valuable in helping this, both in their role as prebiotics, but also due to the fact that they are from the same environment and therefore help remind us of our natural state. Also, there is a lot of information in these foods and many micronutrients which benefit our tissues but also the flora.

Absorption and digestion

The gut flora can optimise the release of calories from oligosaccharides that our own digestive enzymes cannot breakdown; they can also modulate absorption. A healthy gut flora will metabolise dietary fibre into short chain fatty acids. If the gut flora is absent, an animal will need a higher calorific intake to maintain their body weight and will be more prone to vitamin deficiencies especially vitamins B and K.

The brain-gut-microbiota axis and neuroendocrinology

We saw earlier that neurological diseases such as Alzheimer's and Parkinson's give rise to signs in the gut complex as well as the nervous system. We also postulated that there is feedback in both directions. This means that the microflora may be involved in the regulation of neurological function, or more properly neuroendocrine function via the vagus nerve connections and the HPA. The HPA is involved in the initiation of the adrenal stress response. In animals with a reduced or absent gut flora, a mild stress produces an exaggerated release of corticosteroids and ACTH. Re-colonisation of the gut flora helped to normalise the response. It has also been suggested that healthy development of the gut flora in early life is necessary to ensure normal development of the HPA axis; early administration of antibiotics, high-stress environments, inappropriate weaning may impede this; but we can always remediate this through appropriate probiotics, prebiotics and herbs. As it has been shown, treatment with probiotics will enable the stress response to normalise. It is also possible that the gut flora are involved with pain perception since *Lactobacillus* strains can induce the expression of opioid and cannabinoid receptors in the intestinal epithelial cells and can mimic morphine in promoting analgesia.

Both anxiety and memory dysfunction have been shown to be treatable by probiotics or other interventions via the gut microbiota. From this information, we start to get a hint that some of our nervines and endocrine herbs may actually be feeding into this place as well as other parts of our organism.

Also, the brain can alter the gut flora. The brain can induce the secretion of signalling molecules into the gut lumen which can affect gut motility, gut secretion and gut permeability. This causes a change in the gut environment which will in turn alter the population size and composition. Stress has also been shown to make the gut lining more permeable so that bacteria and antigens can cross into the mucosal layer and initiate an immune response that will alter the composition of the gut flora. Acute stress will induce changes in permeability, alter mast cell behaviour and induce high secretion of various substances involved in immune response—leaky gut. Adrenaline and noradrenaline have been shown to show an ability to promote the growth of E. coli strains (both benign and pathogenic). Prenatal stress and postnatal trauma such as maternal separation have been shown to have an effect too. We can start to realise that the gut flora and the whole complex can have a significant effect in many conditions from dementia to autism to IBS and beyond.

Connections with the vagus nerve (pneumogastric nerve or cranial nerve x)

So here is the next connection, the one that links the BGM axis, HPA axis and the heart/parasympathetic axis to make the vertical and horizontal cross axes.

The vagus nerve is the major part of our parasympathetic nervous system, and 80–90% of its fibres are concerned with taking information/messages from the viscera to the brain rather than the other way around. It connects up various parts of us from our ears to our lungs (this is why we cough when we clean out our ears with a cotton bud), to our heart, to our intestines. The one part it does not connect to is the adrenals.

The vagus nerve has a centre which is stimulated by tastes, so when we eat wild foods and herbs it is getting a lot of info about being in Nature (all our brains prefer natural stimulation). It is probable that this stimulation does not just occur via the taste receptors on our tongues; there are similar receptors throughout our GIT and also in other places such as our respiratory system and our spine.

What this also means is that pain, disease and/or stress in quite widely separated parts of the body can affect other regions. What it also means is that we can utilise this knowledge to bring about amazing therapeutic effects with our plant medicines but also with some simple ways of activating the parasympathetic flow through the vagus nerve to treat for example IBS, colitis, sinusitis, neurogenic coughs, supraventricular tachycardia, atrial fibrillation, heartburn—the list is quite remarkable. A commonly reported symptom is a sensation of a lump in the throat accompanied by digestive disturbance; this is due to the adrenal response in the nerves of the oesophagus giving a choking feeling—that's why CST and nervines will help to resolve this, as will herbs that work on vagal tone and parasympathetic balance.

The investigations of the gut could be expanded on much further and longer. However, we will now move onto how this impinges on our relationship with our plant allies.

Re-evaluating the mode of actions of various herbs in light of this.

- Resins are known to be anti-inflammatory and increase leucocytosis; by doing this in the GIT, it would promote a more systemic reduction in inflammation, especially in the case of atopic reaction elicited by food and connected to leaky gut.
- Repairing the gut wall gives a better sense of integrity and restores boundaries, e.g., *Calendula, Filipendula, Achillea, Camellia, Cinnamomum, Mentha, Alchemilla, Rubus*.
- Bitters—we know that many bitters have a reputation as nervines and specifically for the treatment of depression. So *Gentiana lutea* contains xanthones (bitter substances which have been described as having an MAOI effect), but perhaps bitters act on the gut-brain as well as the CNS to elicit these effects.
- *Mentha x piperita* definitely works on vagal tone, as well as exerting a spasmolytic effect; probably most volatile oil-rich herbs do.
- Cyanogenic glycosides work on vagal tone.

In addition to the central digestive tube from the mouth down to the anus we have the additional digestive organs; the liver and gallbladder and the pancreas.

The gall bladder releases the bile produced in the liver to help us digest fatty foods and helps us be decisive. The liver is very much to do with digestion, manufacture and processing wastes. As well as helping break down waste products of digestion, it deals with our emotional waste as well. The liver can become stagnant if it does not feel able to process all that is coming it. It can become overburdened with all the stresses of modern life. Liver cleansing can help to release this. The emotion associated with the liver is anger or determination, which is the energy to change the things we do not like but also to change our attitude to things when necessary. If we are not flexible like supple tree branches, if we are too rigid, then it can lead to a build-up of rage and anger rather than positive energy for change.

The pancreas produces pancreatic juices, an alkaline secretion containing enzymes the continue the digestion of proteins, carbohydrates and fats and also produces the hormones insulin and glucagon to balance blood sugars. It produces several other hormones; pancreatic polypeptide, somatostatin, secretin, incretin, gastrin, and amylin. Pancreatic function can be affected by stress and the effects of adrenalin on the HPA. The emotion of worry is associated with the spleen/pancreas and it can be thrown out of balance when we are ungrounded and lose our connection to the Earth which can make us crave sugar and sweet things.

Classifications of herbs beneficial to the GIT

Although all herbs and foods can have a therapeutic effect on the guts, there are some classes that are seen as having particularly useful benefits.

Bitters stimulate the production of bile in the liver and its release from the gall bladder. They can also stimulate the release of pancreatic juices. These two effects help to encourage healthy digestion, and so bitters are traditionally taken before eating (e.g. vermouth, Campari, suzé-all combinations of bitters, aromatics and alcohol) or after in the form of coffee, almonds, dark chocolate. Bitters also help to engage the enteric nervous system by mechanisms yet to be clearly elucidated and understood; it is possibly via the taste receptors. In addition, they are cooling, clearing and help to drain stagnant energy in the body and move the circulation. Hepatics, cholagogues, choleretics.

Arctium lappa, Artemisia sp., Azadirachta indica, Berberis vulgaris et aquifolium, Calendula officinalis, Carbenia benedicta, Carduus marianus, Coffea arabica, Chicorium intybus, Citrus aurantium fructus, Commiphora molmol, Curcuma longa, Cyanara scolymus, Erythrea centaurium, Gentiana lutea, Glycyrrhiza glabra, Humulus lupulus, Matricaria recutita, Marrubium vulgare, Rumex crispus, Stachys betonica/officinalis, Taraxacum officinale, Theobroma cacao, Urtica dioica, Verbena officinalis, Teasel.

Mucilages act as demulcents, soothing inflammation in the gut wall. They also act as prebiotics for the development of a healthy gut flora. Mucopolysaccharides are a class of mucilage's found particularly in roots, seaweeds and mushrooms that are particularly valuable as immunomodulants. Seaweeds, *Althea officinalis, Avena sativa, Hordeum vulgare, Inula helenium, Malus sp., Plantago lanceolata/major/psyllium, Pulmonaria officinalis, Tilia europea, Ulmus falva.*

Aromatics and carminatives are plants rich in essential oils that relax the guts so that they can absorb food and digest it more easily. Some probably also have a relaxing effect on the vagus nerve. They are often warming, encouraging the circulation to the guts to aid digestion.

Anethum graveolens, Angelica archangelica, Citrus aurantium and other species, Foeniculum vulgare, Humulus lupulus, Lavandula angustifolia, Matricaria recutita, Melissa officinalis, Mentha x piperita, Ocimum basilicum et sanctum, Origanum vulgare, Pimpinella anisum, Piper nigrum, Rosa damascena, Rosmarinus officinalis, Salvia sp., Thymus vulgaris, Tilia x europea, Zingiber officinale.

Cyanogenic glycosides work on the vagus nerve to relax the digestive system, heart and respiratory system. *Prunus serotina, Achillea millefolium, Sambucus nigra.*

Spasmolytics/antispasmodics.

Citrus aurantium flos, Matricaria recutita, Mentha x piperita, Valeriana officinalis, Viburnum opulus.

Nervines for the guts are mainly the aromatic and bitter herbs.

Anti-inflammatories mucilage rich and anthocyanin-rich and *Scutellaria baiacalensis,* resin herbs

Anthocyanin-rich *Sambucus nigra fructus, Vaccinium myrtillus.*

Resins promote leucocytosis and encourage healing and reduction of inflammation. *Boswellia sp., Commiphora species, Curcuma longa.*

Sour astringents *Hibiscus flos,* most summer berries, lemon, rosehips, sumac.

Astringents help to heal mucous membranes in the gut.

Achillea millefolium, Alchemilla vulgaris, Camellia sinensis, Cinnamomum zeylanicum/verum, Mentha x piperita, Rubus idaeus.

Anthroquinones are irritant laxatives; they stimulate peristalsis in the gut. They are not suitable for spasmodic constipation and need the presence of bile to work properly, so a bitter needs to be included in the formula. A carminative is also usually included to prevent cramping.

Rheum, Rhamnus, Rumex, Senna.

- Serotonin: *Urtica dioica* and tryptophan-rich food.
- Saponins: *Glycyrrhiza.*
- Essential fatty acids: walnuts, hemp seed, flax seed, blackcurrant seed, oil raspberry seed oil, borage/starflower oil, rosehip oil and also evening primrose oil.

Immune modulants are herbs and foods that help balance and enhance immune function. There are many classes of immunomodulants and since 70% of our immune function is down to our gut flora most herbs that enhance gut health are immune modulant.

Glucosinolates are the mustard oils. They are immunomodulant and stimulate digestion in small doses. In larger doses, they can be emetic.

Brassica sp., Armoracia rusticana, Capsella bursa-pastoris.

Tuning into the guts, the forgotten continent

For many people their abdominal region is a forgotten continent, a place never visited, the route to listening to this most fundamentally important brain which has been forgotten. It is a place of wonders and may hold some very friendly demons who can help us negotiate the world.

So, we can take time to listen to the stories of our guts.

Take time to ground yourself as we have with each exercise. Remember that for the journey to the guts it is especially important to be grounded as this is our place of internal composting and the places of our roots. Ground and centre yourself with some deep breaths. Let the tension flow out of the body. Remind yourself of the image of the surface that one is sitting on is the supportive, protective, loving hands of the Earth.

Then breathe through your heart since this is the first place to visit on the journey to the guts back to our centre of entrainment. From that place, we can reach down into the guts with a translator if it is a forgotten region. Remember to approach this from that pure, innocent child energy we have explored and remember that the guts are truly a region of gestalt, so the inner child is a great ally. Now bring your focus into your abdomen. Listen to the tissues of the belly, the stomach, the small intestines, the bowel. How do they feel, are they relaxed or constricted or asleep? Are they toned or tense? How are your gut flora, are they a happily balanced ecosystem or do they need something from you—more water, more fibre, more appreciation, some massage, some bitters or aromatic teas? Are the bowels holding onto old emotional junk or physical junk? Take time to listen and tune in. You may find the guts responding by relaxing and releasing wind or gurgling loudly, that is fine. The guts may decide they need to release other things too. A great time to do this exercise is between 5 and 7 am which is the time of day for the large intestine meridian, and this can help to establish a healthy bowel motion first thing in the morning. Anyhow, once you have finished talking to the guts thank them.

Remember to thank them for the work they do before and after your meals too if you feel like it, or if they seem to want that.

The kidney/adrenal complex and urinary system; into the deep, dark waters

Once there was a young person who lived in a small village in a kind and loving but rather fearful family. The village was a safe place to grow up, surrounded by a fence and was at the edge of a big wild forest. Villagers would not venture far into the forest because it was a wild, uncivilised place full of all sorts of animals and plants. This young person was counselled never to venture far into the forest and never ever to stray from the path. But, as we know, sometimes those words of caution excite curiosity. So, one day the young person ventured into the forest to pick some berries for the annual jam making meitheal that the village held each harvest time to prepare stores for the winter. On this particular day though the curiosity overcame the warnings; they walked further into the forest, and before they knew it they had strayed from the well-worn path, seduced by a thicket of beautiful ripe berries lying deeper into the wild. And of course, they started to eat the berries, they started to smell and taste the plants, they listened to the scurryings in the undergrowth and the song of the birds. As they listened and smelt, tasted, looked and touched they felt a stirring in their heart and soul, a remembering of the time when the ancestors had lived deep in the forest, before the fear crept in and they moved into villages surrounded by fences. The wildness within awoke, and they found themselves feeling part of the forest; they realised that they were part of a much bigger community of beings; they came home. When it got dark, they lay down under a large spreading tree and fell asleep lulled by the lullaby of the breeze blowing through its leaves and awoke to the chorus of the birds in the morning. It is not clear how many days they spent walking through the woods, drinking wild water from the stream, eating wild food from the plants but they found themselves. Anyhow, after some time—was it days, weeks, years?—they reached a place where the trees started to thin out, and they found themselves emerging from the forest onto the shores of a large lake. When they looked, they could see a beautiful island in the middle of the lake and on that island they could see a grove of the most magnificent apple trees laden with golden apples, apples that shone with vitality, apples that their soul told them were the most glorious food, full of love and wisdom, of universal communion. They longed to get to the island and pick an apple. But when they looked there was no boat, no way of travelling over the water. When they looked the water looked deep, dark, cold, probably full of all manner of monsters that might devour them. Then they looked up at the island again; the apples pulled a song of longing deep from their soul. What to do? Turn back into the forest and return to the village? Stay on the shores of the lake filled with longing? Or perhaps step into the waters and see what lay beneath? Or perhaps dive into the waters, overcoming the fear? So, this particular young person listened to their indigenous soul and plunged into the water. As they swam deep in the water they saw that there were indeed many unfamiliar beings, but although they were different they were not monsters and demons, they could become friends and so after what seemed like a long swim, or was it a short one, they found themselves reaching the shore of the island and emerged out of the deep dark waters. They climbed the gentle slope to the apple trees, plucked an apple, remembering to give thanks to the tree which radiated pure love and ate the fruit; the most wonderful bliss, that ecstatic feeling of connecting into the Universe rushed into them, and they lay beneath the tree, their heart singing. Now again there was a choice to be made. Would they stay in that place communing with the trees in love? Would they ask to take some of the fruit and plunge back through the waters to return through the forest to bring this gift back to the village? Would they only go back as far as the forest? Would they return to the village with the gift, hoping to lead the way through the forest to this place for others, how would the villagers receive them?

The young person had many choices to make, and really the end of the story depends on what decisions they made; the story never ends, it is our life journey.

The urinary system does the work of filtering the blood, balancing the fluids, salts and water-soluble wastes in our body and eliminating water and wastes. The kidneys are intimately involved in balancing and equilibrating our internal environment to our external environment on a physiological level. On an emotional level, they tell us when we find our external environment stressful or scary and filter out some of our emotional waste as well. When we are under stress, we often experience the need to pass water lots.

They also produce erythropoietin which helps us to create more red blood cells, particularly at high altitude when there is less oxygen available or if there is bleeding. Erythropoietin acts on the bone marrow. Erythropoietin increases the red blood cell count and therefore allows more oxygen to reach the muscles in order to do their work. It is probable that the increased synthesis of erythropoietin that occurs with living at high altitude or other causes of hypoxia (low oxygen levels) is mediated by the skin. The skin cells detect the lack and reduce blood flow to the kidneys. We can also produce erythropoietin in the brain if the levels of oxygen there become low; this protects the neural tissue of the brain from damage.

Calcitriol is the active form of vitamin D. It is formed in the kidneys from calciferol synthesised in the skin with UV exposure and from vitamin D in the diet; the form produced by sun exposure seems to be able to be stored in the body during the dark months, whereas ingested forms are more labile. The calciferol produced in the skin is converted in the liver to 25[OH] vitamin D which is then transported to the kidneys and converted to calcitriol with the help of the parathyroid hormone. So, once again, there is an intimate interaction between the skin and the kidneys. Calcitriol helps the cells of the intestines to absorb calcium from our food and may also have an effect on our intestinal flora to facilitate this absorption; it also acts on our bones to affect the absorption and resorption of calcium from the stores in these tissues, so once again there is an interaction between the kidneys and the bones. Calcitriol is also known as 1,25-hydroxyvitamin D. and has been shown to play an important role in our immune function. It stimulates the differentiation of cells and decreases proliferation and therefore reduces cell mutations that can lead to cancer. It acts as a modulator of the immune system, enhancing our innate immunity and may reduce the development of autoimmune disease; most cells of the immune system have vitamin D receptors, and macrophages sometimes convert 25(OH) vitamin D into the active form in the same way the kidneys do. The cells of the Islets of Langerhans in the pancreas, the ones that secrete insulin, also have vitamin D receptors. Vitamin D may also decrease the risk of developing hypertension since it helps to prevent inappropriate activation of the renin-angiotensin system described below.

The kidneys also monitor and balance blood pressure. If the blood pressure drops too low the kidneys secrete a substance called rennin which splits angiotensinogen in the blood to make angiotensin 1; this is further split by an enzyme secreted by the blood vessels to produce angiotensin II. Angiotensin II closes down the capillary beds by constricting the walls of the arterioles and stimulates the proximal tubules of the kidneys to reabsorb sodium. Angiotensin II also works on the adrenal cortex, stimulating the release of aldosterone which in turn causes further reabsorption of sodium and water. This hormone also acts on the heart to increase the strength of the heartbeat and stimulates the pituitary to release a hormone called vasopressin of which we shall learn more later. All of the actions result in an increase in blood pressure.

The adrenal glands sit atop the kidneys forming a complex situated in the lower back, a region associated with how supported and loved we feel in our life, or how isolated and fearful we are about our security.

Stress means bending out of shape; the degree depends on the force exerted and the material being bent. Stress is anything that places demands on the human organism. Not all stress is bad. For example, going for a run places demands on our body, but yields a positive result. It is only if this is carried to excess that it becomes negative. It is only when we are subjected to too much stress or if we have too little stimulation (i.e. sensory deprivation) that problems arise. Positive stress can lead to achievement. We would normally call these challenges. Indeed, one useful coping mechanism is to change the concept of a problem into a challenge. Negative stress affects us emotionally, mentally and physically. Mental and emotional stress leads to negative thoughts and therefore into negative perceptions and belief systems. These in turn can lead to physical symptoms. When the body is under stress, it produces more acid which causes cell irritation leading to inflammation, tissue breakdown and finally to physical disease as the body becomes congested and cannot eliminate all the toxins produced.

When we are exposed to stress, certain physiological responses called the fight-or-flight responses occur, although it should more properly be called fight, flight, freeze or fun (since it is the same response when we are excited by positive stress it is just that the emotional tone is different). Our bodies become ready to run away or to fight, or to play possum; at least that is the way men respond. This was all very well when the threat was a sabre-toothed tiger but is not so appropriate when dealing with the bank manager, an angry boss/client, sitting an exam, or getting stuck at the traffic lights. There is no occasion to burn off the hormones and nutrients which are released into the system, and this leads to the feelings of exhaustion, headaches and so on that occur after a heavy day, unless we start to run away from people or punch them on the nose. However, in 2000, Shelley Taylor and her research team published a paper called 'Biobehavioural responses to stress in females: tend-and-befriend, not fight-or-flight'.

In the introduction, they point out that:

'The human stress response has been characterised, both physiologically and behaviourally, as "fight-or-flight". Although fight-or-flight may characterise the primary physiological responses to stress for both males and females, we propose that, behaviourally, females' responses are more marked by a pattern of "tend-and-befriend". Tending involves nurturant activities designed to protect the self and offspring that promote safety and reduce distress; befriending is the creation and maintenance of social networks that may aid in this process. The biobehavioural mechanism that underlies the tend-and-befriend pattern appears to draw on the attachment-caregiving system, and neuroendocrine evidence from animal and human studies suggests that oxytocin, in conjunction with female reproductive hormones and endogenous opioid peptide mechanisms, may be at its core. This previously unexplored stress regulatory system has manifold implications for the study of stress'.

This shows that the majority of what is written about our stress responses is based on only half the human population and we need to consider this carefully.

Short-term or lower level stress causes the release of adrenaline, also known as epinephrine or adrenaline, from the adrenal glands and from some of the neurons of the central nervous system. Adrenaline acts as both a hormone and a neurotransmitter. It acts on many tissues of the body to facilitate running away or fighting, although an excess can lead to panic, scattered thinking and complete collapse (the possum effect). Adrenaline acts on the heart to increase the heart rate, the lungs to increase breathing rate, it relaxes the bronchi to facilitate this but constricts the smooth muscles of the small blood vessels to divert blood away from the skin to the skeletal muscles and vital organs; it also facilitates the release of sugars and fats to improve energy production throughout the body. Some adrenaline is released in pleasurable activities; it is also released during childbirth, but its effects are dose-dependent. Often adrenaline and endorphins are released at the same time and some people become addicted to their endogenous adrenaline and endorphins seeking out extreme sports or excessive levels of exercise and the like. Continual exposure to high levels of adrenaline can lead to circulatory conditions such as Raynaud's, digestive problems (chronic diarrhoea or constipation or IBS as the blood is diverted away from the digestive system), stress incontinence, and other urinary problems, hyperventilation, high blood pressure, blood sugar and blood fat imbalances. High levels of adrenaline can also cause an oesophageal spasm causing a sensation of a lump in the throat as well as various unexplainable gastric pains and disturbances.

Higher levels of stress cause the release of cortisol. Small increases in cortisol are beneficial since it can help to release more energy from tissues stores, help heighten memory functions, give a small boost to the immune system, reduce our sensitivity to pain and help maintain homeodynamic balances. Cortisol levels increase during pregnancy, and we have a diurnal pattern of cortisol production; it should usually peak about 30 minutes after rising and make us feel hungry (lack of appetite in the morning is an indication of cortisol insufficiency from adrenal exhaustion or burnout), with another peak in the afternoon.

However, long-term stress (when we do not get the opportunity to return to the relax, restore repair mode) leads to negative effects of cortisol such as impaired cognitive function, underactive thyroid function, blood sugar imbalances (hyperglycaemia, type II diabetes), decreased bone density (osteopenia and osteoporosis), large quantities of dilute urine passed with frequency or urgency, damage to the hippocampus that results in impaired learning and inhibition of stored information from the memory, decreased muscle tissue as it is broken down to provide more energy, raised blood pressure or sometimes very low blood pressure due to the vasovagal response, reduced immune function, inflammatory diseases, poor wound healing, raised cholesterol, heart disease, strokes, metabolic syndrome, deposition of fat in the abdomen; menstrual irregularity or infertility in the female, impotence or infertility in the male, thinning of the skin and skin infections such as tinea or impetigo, acne, hirsutism in women, easy bruising; constant high levels of this hormone lead to many of the health problems we see around us today in the West. Sometimes the body will attempt to redress the vagal balance by inducing an extremely strong response from the vagal parasympathetic system; this may show as outright syncope or fainting, or may present with the prodromal symptoms of nausea, light-headedness, tinnitus, sensation of extreme heat accompanied by sweating, uncomfortable sensation in the heart with or without palpitations and tachycardia, fuzzy thoughts, the inability to form words, stuttering, weakness, visual disturbances such as bright lights, tunnel vision, extreme weakness due to the drop in blood pressure and lack of blood to the brain.

The adrenal glands can become so depleted after a period of long-term stress that they lose the ability to produce sufficient levels of this cortisol. This can lead to weight loss, malaise, general weakness, loss of appetite, nausea and vomiting, diarrhoea or constipation, postural hypotension, low blood sugar, hyper-pigmentation of areas exposed to sunlight, areas that are pressed on such as around the joints, mucous membranes, the conjunctivae and recent scars.

Constant fear will lead to depression; emotional, mental, immuno-logical. It will also result in inflammatory disease for which steroids may be given. Alternatively, non-steroidal anti-inflammatory drugs may be used (prescribed or OTC); chronic use and overuse to suppress inflammation and reduce pain (which is our body's way of signalling that we are unduly stressed) damages … our kidneys.

Fear is a primary emotion. It tells us when we do not feel safe; it lets us know that there is danger. Along with anger and grief it has negative connotations within our culture, and we need to release these; we need to be able to speak out when we do not feel safe; a true warrior is not someone without fear (that is a fool), but rather one who faces fear and has the courage to move through it; someone who knows that the fear itself cannot hurt you. We need to be willing to feel the emotion and know which part of us feels it and work out how to make ourselves feel safe again, how to survive through the experience, how to overcome it. A coward is not someone who feels fear; it is someone who allows fear to control them; someone who feels no fear may well be a fool since the world has many dangers.

Our most primal fear is the fear of not surviving; many things can challenge this, and one of the arenas in which it may be played out is in that of intimacy. We fear intimacy because it requires total vulnerability; vulnerability means we may not survive. Unless we overcome this conundrum, it is difficult to achieve intimacy, since at some level we may believe that it may lead to oblivion, and the ego may tell us to avoid intimacy and connection, to avoid community in case we lose our individual identity in that place of connection. It takes a degree of emotional maturity to negotiate with this part of our inner council to move into a more intimate relationship with our communities—those within us, our human community, the wider community of species that we share our ecosystem with.

Our primary fear of death may also be played out in fear of being ridiculed for being different for truly expressing our core self within the monoculture of Western civilisation as we may be ostracised or even killed for being different. This fear is understandable given the history of colonising people who seek to make everything the same as themselves, who actively seek out those who are different and force them to conform or be killed. The playing out of this game may be more subtle in modern times in 'civilised' societies, but the root fear and the root persecution are still the same.

The fear of death is an interesting one. The only thing that is certain when we are born is that we are incarnated as mortals, that we will die one day. Our culture has moved into a place where immortality is being sold as a false dream. Suffice to say at the moment that if we decide to accept our mortality and therefore to live each moment fully, to step onto our soul path and live our expression of spirit fully many fears dissolve. The fears that remain can be faced from a more heart-cantered place where we walk naked into fear, into life, able to be transparent about who we are. It can be challenging, but it is a far more vital existence. Instead of just existing we live.

We live in a culture of fear. This is not natural. In order for the capitalist system to exist it needs drones; the best way to create drones is to make people very afraid, to remove their security about their primary needs and their ability to fulfil these (food, shelter, medicine, community), to make them believe that they are dependent on the State or others for these primary rights. We should not be born fearful but actually a lot of people are born fearful, either because of exposure to high levels of stress hormones via their mother's bloodstream, or because they received the message in the womb that they were not wanted; womb experiences have a very big impact on the kidney energy and adrenals, to be born already immersed in fear, flight and fight is not natural. We are fed fear by our culture about some of our most basic rights; the health care system has become an industry trying to punt investigations, surgery, pharmaceuticals, tests and therefore needs us to believe that we are not intelligent enough to understand our own bodies and our health. The agricultural and food processing industries teach us to be afraid about our food—food security, inability to grow sufficient, toxins in it, afraid that we are not intelligent enough to understand what to eat. Food is love, not fear. We are taught to be afraid of Nature, that it is full of pathogens trying to kill us, dangerous plants that want to poison us; we are part of Nature not separate from the rest of the community of beings on this planet. We are afraid of all the psychopaths; it is sensible to be scared of psychopaths, but their number has been greatly exaggerated by the media. We are afraid of being bullied at school, of being ridiculed for not achieving academically, of not fitting in, of not being 'normal'. We are afraid about the security of our homes—all those burglars waiting to break in, the banks taking them from us, tempests and floods destroying them. Religion may hold us in a place of fear and shame—we are told we are born sinful, we sin all our lives, so many things are bad, and God is very angry at us, and we live in hell, and when we die we might not get to heaven. We can live in heaven here and now if we see through the illusions and the fear. Or we can live in fear and experience hell on earth.

But above all, we are taught to be afraid of stepping into our power and of anything that is not 'normal'. Since only the material, the mechanistic, the mundane is 'normal' in mainstream culture that means that so much becomes frightening. We are not just physical beings, and we do not just sense the physical. Small children will naturally talk to plants and animals and 'imaginary' friends'—this is ordinary and natural. But society laughs at it and claims it is fantasy. When small children are scared of the dark, of certain people, they are often told their fears are unfounded and to 'be brave'; they are discounted, their experiences are discounted rather than them being encouraged to trust their own feelings, to speak out their fears and seek support from their community of carers. When we are told this, we may store all that fear and terror in our kidneys in order to survive, hiding all that emotional energy so that we will not be annihilated. This means that we shut down parts of ourselves that tell us when we need to feel fear and act to take ourselves into a safer place; when that happens, we buy into all sorts of unnatural ideas. If a child is sensitive to emotional and energetic information (which they all are) so often, they are told to grow out of it. They are not mentored through it and taught healthy ways of staying safe. We tell our children to run away from psychopaths and to tell if they are being bullied, but do we tell them to ask for protection when they are being bullied on a psychic level when people try to scare them or to steal their power? So many people experience adrenal fatigue because they allow other people to feed on their energy, drain their kidneys because they learned this behaviour early in childhood in order to survive! For so long our culture has ignored so much of our emotional and spiritual selves. So, people stuff huge parts of themselves into the bag as Robert Bly puts it, or experience what is called soul loss in some cultures. They do what they need to survive the domestication that is forced on them.

Our culture continually telling us to be afraid means many people are stuck in the Hypothalamic-Pituitary-Adrenal axis fear, flight or fight response, we have been taught to believe this is our natural state; it is not. There is plenty of evidence within the natural world that animals are evolved to spend most of their time in the parasympathetic cordial axis or Relax, Restore, Repair, Rejuvenate and that the adrenal response is supposed to provide the energy to deal with crises and then calm down again; look at a cat, or a cow, an antelope, a lion, they all spend a great deal of their life relaxing if they are living in their natural environment. Humans are supposed to do the same.

Often, when an animal has experienced a fright, it will find a safe place and then shake or re-enact the trauma, this allows the body to release the trauma. I have seen this happen for people having craniosacral treatment, or other unwinding medicine and we often jerk or shudder as we are relaxing to go to sleep which is a similar practice happening spontaneously. Sometimes shaking can also be a receiving of healing and vitality or awen from the rest of Nature; the way we get all goose bumps and shivery when we see a beautiful sunset, get a hug from our beloved or a loved one, or find pleasure coursing through our bodies when we hear music that touches us deeply, eat soul food, smell a rose. Shaking and shivering is about getting the energy moving, we are part of the flow of energy, flowing in and through and out; energy flows like water in a healthy system, and the urinary system is intimately involved in the flow of water (and therefore energy) through our bodies.

Shame is a taught emotion, a fear of being yourself, or of being truly seen. Guilt is different, although it is often a taught emotion too, and it is probably a mixture of sad and scared about the things we have done. These are the emotions that create deep dark secrets. Deep dark secrets can crystallise into pathology. They cause inertia, lack of mobility, cold tissue depression.

Jealousy is due to a perception/belief of lack and of not liking self. It leads people to want to steal another's power/gifts/light; it leads people to want to wound others or what is precious to them; to vandalise the glowy bits or even to try and steal people for themselves.

Fear and grief can be intimately connected; so often part of the grieving process involves feelings of fear. There can be a lot of fear around love too—am I good enough, what if love turns to despising or rejection? What if I am unlovable, what if I am only loved conditionally? This is an epidemic in our society. Let's be clear—love is always unconditional; if it is conditional it is not love, it is manipulation. Yet, as we grow, so often we are told 'I will love you if ...' And so, our view of what love is becomes warped.

Fear can also be connected with anger; we get angry about being scared, especially if this has been a calculated act by a perpetrator. We are also told not to get angry when people scare us but isn't that what the whole fear flight or fight apex is about—we get scared, we decide whether to run away (really scared) or get angry and stay and fight? And when we do react in those ways, we are fed shame; be afraid of being yourself and acting in a natural way. And so, we lose a part of ourselves, and then we grieve, except that is not 'normal' either, we grieve, we get depressed, we experience sorrow and sadness, and then our culture wants us to suppress that grieving process too. Of course, we are morally responsible for choosing an appropriate part of ourselves to step forward when we are scared, one that does not externalise our inner turmoil and spread the inner panic.

Any imbalance in the kidney-adrenal complex will also tend to affect the bladder energy; in several systems of traditional medicine the kidney and bladder are associated with water, those deep dark waters of emotion we have to swim through to reach the golden apples. Water is associated with our emotions; water is affected by the cycles of the moon as evidenced by the effects the moon has on the tides; ask anyone who works in a psychiatric ward, and they will tell you that the most challenging time at work is just around the full moon.

Courage is the transcendence of fear; the fear does not go away, but we learn to recognise that it is a warning system that tells us we need to act, to bring forward the still small voice that overcomes the panicked adrenal response, the one that calmly says we can work through this. We find ourselves becoming comfortable with the idea that the world is a dangerous place and we can keep ourselves safe in it, or deal with it.

Love is the cure for fear

So how do we redress this imbalance, how do we move from the place of fear into the place of relaxation? How do we ensure that we get to do the relax, restore, repair, rejuvenate place?

One approach is fear management; developing coping and survival skills, tucking the fear away in the back of our mind, in our adrenals, wherever. We get through. But it's supposed to be better than mere survival and existence. Can we move to transcend fear?

We produce another hormone called oxytocin from our pituitary gland, and this has been called the hormone of love, the trust hormone, the empathy hormone or the morality hormone by various authors as research has uncovered information showing it to be the hormone of bonding; human beings are social animals and thrive best in support-ive communities. The current cultural cult of the individual, the break-down of community, neighbourhoods and extended families does not serve us well.

All humans produce oxytocin, but oestrogen synergises with oxytocin so that in the woman the effects of it are enhanced and more strongly experienced. Oxytocin does have a physical role to play in facilitating childbirth and expressing milk in nursing, but it also enhances our feel-ings of bonding, helps to reduce bleeding at the placenta after birth and shortens labour by producing strong regular contractions. Adrena-line is also produced during labour to release the energy to meets the demands of what is most certainly hard work and stressful, but it is the balance of these two hormones that is important since too much adrena-line will cause distress to the unborn child, cause contractions to slow, stop, become erratic and lengthen the labour. Oxytocin is the molecule of bonding, nesting, pair bonding, nurturing, protecting and accepting offspring and influences our mate selection; it prevents depression but can cause a degree of emotional lability. Oxytocin acts as both a hormone and as a neurotransmitter. Oxytocin promotes touching, affection and bonding and a single touch will cause levels to rise instantly. It lowers stress-related symptoms, counterbalancing the effects of adrenaline and cortisol and helps us get to the relax, restore, repair place. Repeated doses change the instant effect into long-term benefits; the more oxytocin our bodies produce the stronger response it produces both physically and mentally—we actually produce more oxytocin receptors in our neurons. We are more likely to produce good levels of oxytocin if we stay calm (open our hearts). In a stressful situation, oxytocin can help us to stay calm and be able to work our way through to moving out of danger; it inhibits the fear, flight or fight response in the brain. Oxytocin lowers our blood pressure and protects against heart disease, makes us feel calm and connected to our community (internal, and external) and makes us more curious. It reduces cravings for sugar and other addictions. Because oxytocin increases positive feelings and keeps us calm it facilitates learning. It is the hormone of repair and healing and restoration (physically, mentally, emotionally, spiritually) so helps speed up wound healing and tissue repair in general. Oxytocin is the hormone of sexual receptivity, bonding and reduces impotence. Oxytocin also promotes healthy social behaviour and reduces antisocial behaviour. Exogenous oxytocin cannot be given orally, only by a nasal spray; because this is the only route of administration that allows it to pass the blood-brain barrier.

So, in what ways can we elevate our endogenous oxytocin?

As already mentioned, a single touch will do it; hugs are even better. Giving birth and breastfeeding raise levels but so does child nurturing; men's levels rise when they take care of their children, this includes conversation with eye contact and other meaningful interactions as well as hugs. It is probable that oxytocin levels are raised by any nurturing behaviour in both men and women and that this is a positive feedback loop so that the more you do it, the more you produce, the more nurturing you feel. Oxytocin levels increase five times in both men and women during sex, increasing pair bonding. Levels drop straight after in men though.

Dancing, meditation and laughing all increase our endogenous levels. Being in the community increases it, so spending time in our natural environment and sharing heart space with our pets, the plants, the trees, anything that makes us feel connected and harmonious in our inner or outer community will increase our oxytocin levels. Strangely enough, a lot of these activities also reduce cortisol.

The pituitary also produces vasopressin or anti-diuretic hormone as it reduces urine output and elevates blood pressure. Both men and women make it, but it is synergised by testosterone so that it is potentiated in males. As well as increasing water retention and rising blood pressure it can increase the size of the forehead. Emotionally, it is associated with aggression, territorial and hierarchical behaviour. However, it is also the hormone that bonds males to their mates and their children, to their family, promoting mate recognition, pair bonding, mate guarding as well as sexual arousal, partner recognition and courtship behaviour. Vasopressin also enhances memory. Men experience a spike of vasopressin after sexual intercourse; another role of this hormone is that it creates a feeling of separation, withdrawing back into the cave after intimacy, reclaiming the individual. It elicits dampened emotional responses and more rational behaviour.

Testosterone and oestrogen are produced from the adrenals as well as the gonads.

In the female, oestrogen is predominantly produced from the gonads until menopause. It produces the female secondary sexual characteristics of larger breasts and broader hips. It prevents many degenerative diseases such as osteoporosis and heart disease. It helps improve good sleep quality, sensitivity to odours, general sensory acuity and memory. Oestrogen is associated with female sexual behaviour, neuron growth and improved cognition, more stable moods and a sense of wellbeing. Men produce oestrogen from their adrenals and need some oestrogen to maintain strong bones; men involved in caretaking produce more oestrogen.

Testosterone is produced in the gonads by men and in the adrenals by both sexes. Men produce 10 times more testosterone than women. Testosterone secretion in men depends on gaining a higher place in social order or working hard physically. Women who compete in the job place or engage in hard physical labour are likely to produce more testosterone than those who work in the home as carers. Testosterone produces physical characteristics such as body hair, increased muscle bulk, larger bone structure. Emotionally, testosterone creates a sense of separateness, assertiveness, self-confidence, sex drive (rather than affection), aggression, risk-taking, interest in moving objects (cars, planes and the like), visual-spatial ability. It can also produce anxiety, poor concentration, violent, criminal or psychotic behaviour.

This starts to reveal the connection between the adrenals and reproduction, the survival of the species. If all our steroidal hormone backbones are diverted to producing adrenaline and cortisol from the adrenals, then there are less available to produce the gonad hormones necessary for reproduction.

The Lower Cauldron also contains the sacral plexus, a nerve plexus which is essentially one of our brains connected to the others via the vagus nerve. The sacral plexus is more complex in women than in men since there is a lot more coordination needed for female reproductive function and the plexus is also very involved in how safe and secure we feel. We will explore this in our discussions of the neuroendocrine system when we investigate the Upper Cauldron.

Herbs for kidney/adrenal and urinary system

Salt is not all bad; too little leads to depression, so we need some in our diet; the less refined, the better. We can use salty herbs to strengthen the kidney energy such as seaweeds, nettle, plantain, parsley.

Spasmolytic herbs

Spasmolytic herbs help to relax tension so that fear can be shaken out and more positive feelings shaken in;

Mentha x piperita, Viburnum opulus, Valeriana officinalis, Citrus aurantium flos, Matricaria recutita.

Adaptogens

Adaptogens help to replenish the kidney energy. Some local ones are:

Urtica dioica, Taraxacum officinale, Stachys officinalis, Arctium lappa, Salvia officinalis (short-term), *Borago officinalis, Rosmarinus officinalis, Sambucus nigra fructus.*

Also, some of the exotic ones are great too—*Astragalus, Bacopa, Eleutherococcus, Hydrocotyle, Ocimum sanctum, Panax ginseng, Tabebuia, Schisandra, Withania.*

Warming kidney tonics

Warming kidney tonics such as *Petroselinum, Barosma, Levisticum, Thymus vulgaris.*

Urinary demulcents

Urinary demulcents calm inflammation and heat in the urinary tract and include *Malus* in the form of stewed apple or warm apple juice with some cinnamon added, *Hordeum vulgare* in the form of barley water, *Agropyron repens, Althea officinalis herba*—a cold infusion is best to extract the maximum amount of mucilage, *Plantago lanceolata* and *Plantago major, Zea mays.*

Diuretics

A true diuretic means that more water is passed than has been taken in and there are five types:

1. Increase filtration rate—broom, coffee, tea (less so).
2. Salediuretic or saluretic—sodium and salt not reabsorbed draws water with it. *Taraxacum officinale fol.*
3. Osmosis (*Taraxacum officinale*) by sugars, e.g., mannitol, sorbitol, inositol, *Agropyron repens, Zea mays.*
4. Blocks ADH-alcohol.
5. Volatile oils cause soft irritation of kidney.

Apium graveolens, Petroselinum crispum, Levisticum officinale, Asparagus-asparagine, *Betula pendula, Daucus carota* (whole plant), *Fraxinus excelsior* (fruit and leaves), *Levisticum officinale, Juniperus communis, Taraxacum officinale fol, Crataegus oxycanthoides, Filipendula ulmaria, Urtica dioica, Foeniculum vulgare.*

Betulina, Salix, Apium graveolens, and Filipendula ulmaria all act as diuretics and help to flush out excess acids and nitrogenous waste from the body. They sweet our inner terrain in the same way that they sweeten the soil and act as pioneer plants for other trees and species that require a lower pH soil.

Crataegus sp. and *Achillea millefolium* both act as diuretics by promoting peripheral circulation and moving more blood to the kidneys, having the opposite effect to vasopressin.

Taraxacum officinale fol is a diuretic par excellence which reduces water retention, flushes out acid and also acts as a net potassium supplement, thus supporting the heart as well. When there has been a lot of fear, the heart often becomes insulted, diminished.

CHAPTER NINE

The middle cauldron the emotional being

The Middle Cauldron or Coire Ernmae is known as the cauldron of vocation and motion. It is positioned in the centre of the chest in the heart region. All our life experiences of joy and sorrow cause it to turn and fill so that we can walk our vocational path and in time fill our Upper Cauldron.

The Middle Cauldron is about our connection to our community, our emotional wellbeing and our heart star healing capacity; knowing our life path and following it, centred in our community.

We produce a particular form of energy here which is part of our ecological function; it is the energy of compassion and caring and bonding in the community. We also give, receive and process a lot of our emotional intelligence and information in this cauldron.

The song of our heart star

For most of the existence of the human race, the heart was seen as the seat of the soul and as an organ of perception, reading the heart of the world; the heart receives meanings from the world around us and also sends out meanings to the rest of the web; it is in a conversation whether or not we recognise the fact; recognising the fact can significantly alter the tone and content of the conversation. In many cultures there is an association between the heart and joy being expressed through singing, humming or whistling as one travels through the day; through frequent laughter and giggles, through ease with close proximity to our fellow humans, and with physical touch. In the West, it is not such a common practice to walk into the day singing one's heart song, but it is a beautiful thing to do.

In the West, a shift in the cultural epistemology occurred which caused people to move away from the heart space and become centred in the head. Although some authors suggest it started with the move from a hunter-gather society to an agrarian culture, others suggest that it occurred with the beginning of writing and that it became more concrete when Galileo announced that the Universe was a machine. I suspect that the change in cultural paradigm caused a shift in the way people related to Nature since the Kayapo Indians in Brazil demonstrate that humans are completely capable of carrying out synergistic agriculture, so interwoven with the other species of the region that they live in that initially visiting scientists thought that the complex ecosystem was purely without human intervention, so the agrarian way of life does not cause the shift; and there are examples of cultures with a rich written tradition that still walks in harmony with the Earth, although oral tradition in storytelling does add a richness and flexibility that is not always there in written language; the medicine of storytelling is definitely something that needs to be restored in how we teach our children and students and pass on the knowledge of our forebears. Over a period of time, reductionism became the ruling epistemology in the West, rationalism dominated, and humans came to believe that they were machines, separate from Nature. This does not mean that this became true, but belief systems have knock on effects as we have seen. Once the World has no soul, once we are machines, then we no longer need to have any moral obligation to how we treat our planet or our fellow beings. It was a shift towards dominance by the left neocortex that occurred; this is the part of ourselves that believes that the world is a machine, lifeless, that is focused and analytical; it does not like change and prefers to stick to the old tried and tested conventional way of doing anything; it is a most valuable part of ourselves. However, when it is the only part of us that we listen to we are truly kyboshed.

William Harvey first described the circulation of the blood and the heart as the pump driving this circulation in 1628; before this, physicians thought that the heart was a producer of heat, cooled by the lungs, whilst the arteries served to cool the blood. During this time anatomists, physiologists and orthodox scientists were moving to the rationalist view that the laws of physics and chemistry were the only way of describing the functioning of life forms, thus reducing us to machines that could be described by analytical thinking and by quantifying or measuring, rather than feeling the meanings and the qualities of who we are. The heart came to be viewed merely as a pump for circulating re-oxygenated blood to the tissues of the body; the soul no longer had a resting place where it belonged. As it came to be believed that the heart had this sole physical function, it was no longer acknowledged as an organ of perception, that receives emotional meanings from the constant stream of information sent out by the Universe, capable of conducting a nonverbal conversation with the rest of the world. Many people do not realise that this is our natural state.

Given that the language of the heart is the imagination, it then became possible to write off the whole imaginal realm as unreal; at best the imaginal is seen as art, poetry, fanciful notions to distract us from the 'real' world, an indulgence, or at worst superstitious, ridiculous, the stuff of childhood and immaturity or quite possibly dangerous magic, occult. The notion of equal importance of spirit and matter, their inseparability, the idea that they are expressions of one and the same thing came to be seen as ridiculous; since spirit could not be measured or quantified by instruments, since it could not be described by the laws of physics and chemistry, since the physical senses of sight, hearing, taste, touch or smell were deemed not to be able to perceive it then it could be written off. The recognition of the invisibles was felt to be fine for mystics, for religious, for eccentric artists and primitive natives but it was most definitely not to be accepted as part of sensible, rational life or thought. Conditions that could not be explained by reductionism were dismissed as hysteria, psychosomatic, fits of the vapours and the like.

In 1964, George Solomon and his co-researchers coined the phrase psychoimmunology to describe the phenomenon that emotional perturbation could adversely affect immune function; the first orthodox recognition that the mind and emotions actually do affect the physical body. In 1975, Robert Adler and Nicholas Cohen took this a step further to coin the phrase psychoneuroimmunology when they conducted experiments demonstrating that the nervous system could affect the immune system. Candace Pert further demonstrated that neuropeptides and neurotransmitters could directly affect the immune system. Recently our endocrine system has been added into this so that the term is now psychoneuroendocrinoimmunology. And so, by the early twenty-first-century scientists were beginning to accept that disease may actually start in the emotions, rather than in the physical realm.

Rupert Sheldrake has touched on the concept of the interconnectedness of all in the material Universe, and Lyn Margolis has described the Earth as an organism. Traditional healers have spoken about this for thousands of years. A lot of the Western diseases are ones that Christine Page describes as being associated with the heart energy—heart disease, high blood pressure, high cholesterol, cancer, hypersensitivities, allergies, autoimmune disease. Researchers have demonstrated that a return to an indigenous lifestyle cannot just reduce symptoms but completely remove them.

In recent times much new information has been discovered about the heart. The heart is not just two pumps working in tandem divided by the central septum. In fact, the heart's pumping action is not sufficiently forceful to drive the blood circulation alone.

The heart as organ of perception and a 'second brain'

The heart contains more neural tissue than the head-brain (60–65% of its cells are neural cells), it has a stronger electromagnetic field (about 5000 times stronger), and it produces neurotransmitters such as dopamine, noradrenaline and acetylcholine. Acetylcholine plays a part in memory, and a lack of it can lead to Alzheimer's disease. How often do those on heart medication develop forms of memory loss or dementia? Our heart is an emotional brain and an organ of emotional perception, it holds emotional memories. This is something that our ancestors always knew.

The electrical field of the heart can be detected 3.3 metres away by machines, but further by living beings, including humans; the field is normally strongest about 30–45 cm away from the body. One can experience the ability to feel this electromagnetic field with a willing volunteer. One of you stands with your arms open wide and the other walks towards them from a distance of a few metres, face-to-face and maintaining eye contact; opening the arms opens the heart field, being face-to-face facilitates heart communication, and eye contact gives a depth of trust; at a certain point there will be a softening of the eyes, and of the face, perhaps a smile or even a giggle. The nerve cells of the heart are involved in the function of the heart but also connect directly to various parts of the triune brain—the amygdala (emotional memories and processing), thalamus (sensory experience), hippocampus (memory, spatial relationships and making sense of sensory inputs from the external environment) and cortex (problem solving, reasoning and learning). This means that information is passed directly between the two organs in both directions; heart cycles will alter the function of the brain and vice versa. The heart makes neurotransmitters in response to the information it gets from the central nervous system both for its own function and to allow communication with the brain.

The heart also has a memory and holds memories; most often those associated with emotional experience and they influence our perception of the world, our consciousness and behaviour. It has been demonstrated that people who receive transplanted hearts often start to display behaviours that were previously not there but were part of the behaviour of the person from whom they received the heart; the receiver of the donated heart may actually find that their likes, dislikes and preferences become altered.

The heart is probably the primary organ of perception—it receives the information from the world and passes it onto the brain. Due to our cultural attitude towards heart perception (the state in which we are born and sit in naturally as children) we are conditioned out of it into relying on the triune brain. However, the triune brain is more a knowledge store and for sorting the information perceived by the heart and our other senses—it excels in analytical processes which may explain why the shift in our epistemology has resulted in an over-reliance on analytical, linear thinking and the elevation of the reductionist rational approach to a supremacy in most realms, including places where such an approach is rather irrelevant such as the arts. Science and analytical thinking, the measuring of things, can be a very valuable tool when applied appropriately, but like a knife or a chainsaw, it can become extremely dangerous when applied inappropriately; they all can be extremely damaging to living beings. There is a need for balance between the value of measuring, of looking at probabilities, of quantitative assessment and the value of sensing the meanings, asking how does it feel, qualitative assessment?

We have already touched on the concept that hearts will communicate with other hearts; they will entrain and synchronise. When hearts synchronise, there is a huge exchange of information. Also, other organs entrain with the heart; this is known as heart coherence. Ary Goldberger, an American cardiologist, discovered that developing heart coherence can reduce blood pressure by 60 points, without any other intervention.

By sitting with a person and getting them to focus on their heart (focus their attention into where their heart physically resides, even imagine breathing in and out through the heart), to really focus until they feel into the natural state of the heart, the point where the breathing slows, a deep breath may be taken, the pulse rate calms and then the blood pressure drops, as simply as this the person reaches into the parasympathetic mode of the nervous system, into a place of relaxation, restoration. Teach the person how to keep it there, anchor it in; simply do this by repetition, repetition, repetition, taking the time to repeat this exercise for a few minutes a couple of times a day or any time one starts to feel tense, get them to embed the information, to habituate to the natural state of heart. It is so simple, it costs nothing, it has no side effects (except an increased tendency to smile, to laugh, to feel bliss and perhaps to cry from time to time), but it requires application. It is possible to get to the point where it can be automatic to switch in and out as one requires, as is appropriate. It is best if you focus on gratitude or love or appreciation when practising heart coherence, and being in a state of innocent perception will help.

The heart starts to beat before the brain is fully formed and the emotional centres of the brain develop before the rational regions—emotion comes before rationalisation; the cells in the forebrain entrain with the heart, perhaps we need to reconsider which is the dominant brain. The heart communicates with the brain through electromagnetic or energetic information, pressure waves or physically, hormones and neurotransmitters (chemically), and through nerve impulses (neurologically).

The heart also produces hormones. An atrial natriuretic factor is produced in the atria. This hormone works on the blood vessels, kidneys, adrenal glands and the brain. It inhibits the release of stress hormones, interacts with the reproductive organs and immune system. Its effect on the kidneys help to regulate body fluid levels, electrolyte balance and blood pressure—homeostasis (or homeodynamis). ANF also affects the level of hormones and neurotransmitters, including renin, noradrenaline, aldosterone, catecholamines, cortisol, vasopressin and dopamine. ANF is stored in dense cellular bodies, with about two and a half times as many in the right side of the heart than the left. As blood is pushed through the aortic valve, the pressure causes the release of ANF into the blood. High blood pressure depletes ANF and reduces the heart's ability to produce it. BNF or brain naturetic factor is produced in the neurons of the heart ventricles and the brain. It causes the secretion of Beta-amyloid precursor protein which protects the neural tissue of the heart and brain against stressors (e.g., toxic levels of glutamate). Since it protects the hippocampus, it improves its function in learning and memory. A c-type naturetic peptide is a heart-produced vessel dilator which also inhibits pancreatic cancer cells. Calcitonin gene-related peptide works with nitric oxide to promote vasodilation and relaxation and anti-proliferative actions; together these hormones help to protect the arteries from atherosclerosis, coronary heart disease and stroke. If inflammatory factors such as prostaglandins, histamine, bradykinin and lactic acid are raised this will trigger the release of CGRP.

These hormones are very much involved in parasympathetic responses and good immune function. A healthy heart makes us relax; relaxing makes the heart healthy. As indigenous people know our true state of being is in the parasympathetic mode—then we are able to truly relax, to read the meanings in the world, to know that the world is an extremely dangerous place and only by relaxing into this can we make it safe because then we can use all our brains—the heart, the gut, the triune brain and know when we need to switch into the adrenal response to give us the burst of energy to fight hard or run away quickly; then we can use all our sensory acuity to feel into the heart of the scenario we are in. We can calm the shrill voice of panic in the heart and be fully present with 360° senses.

Associations with the heart

The heart is often associated with fire or the sun; associations speaking of radiance and of heat; we describe someone who is being passionate as having their heart on fire or an act of compassion as heart-warming.

Three colours are associated with the heart: gold the colour of star shine; green having a view of green Nature out of the window, or spending time out in Nature has been shown to significantly speed recovery from heart surgery; and pink, our culture can have a rather jaundiced or narrow view of the meaning of this colour, more associated with shadow femininity and sentimentality than with unconditional love. Love is not the same as sentimentality; true love can be rather challenging for many people. Love is not romanticism, nor is it sexuality, nor is it intimacy. Love is unconditional and flows out to touch the world. Love shines into dark places to bring those places to consciousness. Love is a powerful energy and defends us. That is why so many plants that work on the heart energy are warrior plants with thorns as well as great beauty. Plants like rose, hawthorn and the bramble which Glennie Kindred describes as helping us with perseverance in love and spirituality. Love demands that we rigorously examine ourselves and admit what our level of moral development is; that we are willing to see what kind of person we are, what kind of people others are, without judgement—love does not judge, it is unconditional, but it does have clear sight. Love can be fierce like the lion; it is strong like the oak.

True love can be frightening in its intensity, its heat, its brightness; the fact that it is unconditional, that it is everlasting, that it is a shining stream of energy transmitted from an open heart, it does not shut up, it is a pure meaning flowing into the information pool of the world.

Fear is sometimes described as the opposite of love, or is it rather the enemy of love: the energy that will strangle and diminish it; the fear of betrayal, the fear of being truly seen, the fear of having no secrets, the fear of stepping fully in to our power, of rejection, of abandonment, the fear of loss of autonomy and of becoming dependent, no longer being independent; the fear of intimacy, of revealing ourselves, the fear of living transparently, the fear of being morally responsible for our own state of consciousness?

M Scott Peck (in his book *The Road Less Travelled*) says that the opposite of love is laziness because love calls us into action and fear moves us into inertia and laziness.

Loving can be painful as one reaches beneath the surface of things and starts to truly see the wounds, the deep interior wounds of one's self, of those around, and the exterior wounds that those cause in the world. Having said that, loving opens us to see the beauty in the world, in ourselves and in others. The experience of such profound beauty that joy bubbles up and bliss ensues. And, as with birth, the pain and the bliss may well be experienced at the same time. Birthing and living are not techniques, they are real scenarios, we cannot act our way through them, mimicking other people's lives and actions, following techniques—well we can, but it is not very convincing. Rather, we find ourselves, our path; we become authentically ourselves, drop the masquerade.

In our culture, heart-centred can be perceived as weak, whereas formerly it was seen as also having the masculine heart warrior (there are also feminine heart warriors). Now masculinity tends to be aligned with the head. It is interesting to see that cardiovascular disease is more prevalent in the gender that has been discouraged out of their heart space. Half of heart disease related deaths are sudden cardiac death. There is a sudden disruption of the electrical activity in the heart; high levels of stress will cause this and can be cumulative. As women move into a more head-centred place, there is a rise in cardiovascular disease within this gender. When boys reach puberty the first organ in their body to start to enlarge is the heart.

The circulation

Our blood connects all the cells of our body together, bringing nourishment, carrying away waste products, hydrating, bringing chemical information in many forms such as hormones, salts, and other nutrients, so it is also a valuable part of the communication systems of our being but originating in the Middle Cauldron. Our blood cells are mainly made in our bones; they are born from our bones and our bones hold the wisdom of our ancestors, so the blood also carries the wisdom and knowledge of our ancestors to each cell of our bodies. The blood and circulatory system also carries the pressure waves generated in the heart out to our tissues and cells; these waves are another form of information about what is happening in the heart. The balance of the composition of the blood is vital to the continued health of our tissues. The body is continually measuring the blood pressure, the balance of water and electrolytes, the pH (acidity/alkalinity), the red blood cells, white blood cells, levels of oxygen and carbon dioxide. There are complex feedback mechanisms to ensure that these factors are held within the healthy limits.

We know that the average adult heart beats 60–90 times per minute, which is about 100,000 times a day. There are about 8 pints of blood being pumped around, so that is about 64 pints being circulated per minute. The length of the blood vessels through which the blood is being pumped is about 60,000 miles. The beating of the heart alters from stroke to stroke according to the information from the internal and external environment so that a healthy heartbeat is not totally regular; there is a conversation going on all the time. Since the heart is not a mechanical pump, it is healthy for it to adapt to all the information it receives as it is working in a non-linear fashion.

When the heart muscle is pumping the blood it twists, turns and squeezes. This generates a flow through the heart that follows a figure of

8 or infinity symbol; a spiral movement. The heart beats and produces waves of pressure that precede the blood flow through the circulatory system. The pressure waves cause expansion of the vessels which produces an electrical voltage. The waves also 'squeeze' the cells of the body which generates an electrical voltage. This means that as well as the blood carrying nutrients to the cells, they also receive this pressure stimulation which causes an electrical response. In the same way that water spirals down the plughole, the blood travels through the vessels in a spiralling motion—it is actually two entwining spirals (comparable with the DNA strands). Different components of the blood travel in different regions of the vortex—the red blood cells are nearer the centre due to being heavier. The lighter platelets are further out. This centrifugal effect means that different components travel at different speeds. The cells themselves also have a spinning motion through the liquid.

Herbs for the heart and circulation

Circulatory stimulants, peripheral

Achillea millefolium, Angelica archangelica, Cinnamomum verum, Curcuma longa, Ginkgo biloba, Myrica cerifera, Piper nigrum, Rosmarinus officinalis, Zanthoxylum, Zingiber.

Central

Armoracia rusticana, Arnica montana, Capsicum minimum, Curcuma longa, Panax ginseng.

Cerebral

Bacopa monnieri, Crataegus oxycanthoides/laevatiga, Ginkgo biloba, Rosmarinus officinalis, Vinca minor, Salvia officinalis.

Cordials/cardiac tonics

Asclepias tuberosa, Cereus grandiflorus, Cinnamomum verum, Coffea arabica, Convallaria majalis, Crataegus oxychanthoides, Cytisus scoparius, Leonorus cardiaca, Ocimum sanctum, Passiflora incarnata, Prunus serotina, Rosa damascena, Rosmarinus officinalis, Theobroma cacao.

Diuretics

Refer to list on page 156.

Anticoagulants

Allium sativum, Asperula odorata, Galium species, Melilotus officinalis, most beans and pulses, essential fatty acids.

Coagulants

Achillea millefolium, Capsicum minimum, Geranium robertianum et maculatum, Medicago sativa, Plantago lanceolata, Quercus robur, Urtica dioica.

Anti-atheroma

Allium sativum, Arnica montana, Ginkgo biloba, Glychyrrhiza glabra, Hydrastis canadensis, Malus sp., Panax ginseng, Tilia x europea.

Hypertensives

Cytisus scoparius, Ephedra sinica, Mentha x piperita, Rosmarinus officinalis (last two are amphoteric).

Hypotensives

Achillea millefolium, Allium ativum, Convallaria majalis, Crataegus oxycanthoides (amphoteric), *Ginkgo biloba, Leonorus cadiaca, Melissa officinalis, Olea europea, Passiflora incarnata, Valeriana officinalis, Viburnum opulus.*

Circulatory relaxants/vasodilators

Lobelia inflata, Mentha x piperita, Vaccinium myrtillus, Valeriana officinalis, Viburnum opulus, Zingiber officinale, all diaphoretics, some bitters.

Blood vessel tonics

Aesculus hippocastanum, Achillea millefolium, Bellis perennis, Calendula officinalis, Crataegus oxycanthoides, Fagopyrum esculentum, Ginkgo biloba,

Hydrastis canadensis, Sambucus nigra fructus, Tilia x europoea, Vaccinium myrtillus, Citrus pith and all flavonoid rich foods and herbs.

Anti-haemorrhagic/styptic

Achillea millefolium, Capsicum minimum, Geranium robertianum, Geum urbanum, Lamium album, Plantago major et lanceolata, Sanguisorba sp., Urtica dioica.
  Potassium rich herbs: *Armoracia rusticana, Taraxacum officinale fol.*
  Calcium-rich herbs: *Valeriana officinalis.*
  Iron-rich herbs: *Petroselinum crispum, Urtica dioica.*
  Folate-rich herbs: *All fresh leafy greens.*
  B_{12} rich herbs Sprouted seeds and beans, mushrooms, seaweeds (especially dulse and nori).

Rubefacients

Allium sativum, Armoracia rusticana, Brassica species, Juniperus communis, Zingiber officinale.
  Diuretics for oedema: *Taraxacum officinale fol.*

Varicosities/phlebotonics

Achillea millefolium, Aesculus hippocastanum, Calendula officinalis, Vaccinium myrtillus, Hamamelis virginiana, Cupressus sempervirens (externally), essential oils of *oleum, Pelargoneum graveolens/x asperum.*

Arrhythmias

Cheiranthus, Cytisus scoparius, Convallaria majalis, Crataegus laevatiga, Achillea millefolium.

Blood builders

Beta vulgaris, Rehmannia, Urtica dioica.

Vagal nerve tonics

Mentha x piperita, Achillea millefolium, Prunus serotina and other herbs containing cyanogenic glycosides.

The foxglove

An open, warm heart. The flowers are the colour of a healthy heart, they are open and to reach the warmth and nectar one must climb in, be willing to immerse one's self in that warm embrace and to comingle. An open heart is *strong* medicine—the more wounded and damaged the heart the smaller the dose needs to be to start with. One must be willing to receive the nectar that is offered, no more, no less and then give thanks and journey on. A strong medicine will not kill unless one takes more than is needed. The Foxglove can protect itself because it knows itself; an open, warm heart is very vulnerable and very strong. It protects itself by knowing itself and by breaking open the walled heart, by thawing the frozen heart, by nourishing with nectar the starved heart. It roots well into the earth. That rosette of leaves anchors it down to Mother Earth. Like all plants, it feeds itself by transmuting Earth, Water, Fire (Sun) and Air into the food it needs and into the medicine it transmits. The more challenges, the stronger its medicine. But the more nourishment, the healthier it grows.

The bee that feeds on the nectar offers something in exchange— it transfers the pollen to other flowers and ensures that the ova are fertilised, that there is healthy reproduction of the foxglove; there is an exchange of good energies—bee and foxglove work together.

There is another part to the story of Foxglove. It used to be used for water retention, dropsy in folk medicine. Then a doctor heard about an old woman who was using it *in combination with about another 12 herbs*, in a complex community medicine for heart disease (the two conditions are related). He rejected the other parts of the formula and isolated the cardiac glycosides and look what happened then—strong plants like these need to be ameliorated by their companions. The original formula was lost/destroyed? Perhaps we need to look at which plants grow comfortably around the Foxglove to discover how to use it safely again. Some plant medicines work well alone; some need to be combined, especially the really strong ones. Psychic dumping, trying to feed one's negativity into another does happen; it is evil. Being willing to say this stops with me and I give it all back is hard work and is strong medicine. Learning to discern what is projection, what is perception is a long journey. Only give out what one would wish to receive. Learn to compost the rest or offer it up as energy to be transmuted is good.

The lungs and grieving

I was not born to be forced. I will breathe after my own fashion.
Henry David Thoreau: On the Duty of Civil Disobedience.

The lungs are an interface with our external environment. During respiration, we breathe in air and draw all the information contained in this medium into our bodies through the nose and mouth. The respiratory circle has three phases—inhalation, exhalation and a short pause. Breathing is one of the most intimate acts we carry out, one of the most intimate sharings; as we breathe, we inhale gases that may have been exhaled only moments previously by another person, animal or plant. It is also one of the most vital; we can survive a couple of days without water, several weeks without food but only a matter of minutes without breathing in oxygen (although pearl divers and yogis have developed ways of going for longer).

As well as containing oxygen, the air that we breathe contains a massive amount of information such as pheromones, volatile substances, aromas, carbon dioxide, nitrogen, argon, traces of other gases and water vapour at variable levels, depending on the local humidity. It contains streams of chemical information released into the atmosphere by all living beings on the face of the planet, as well as chemical information released by industrial processes and combustion. Plants release all sorts of information into the air in the form of gases and volatile compounds; these may be to attract pollinators (the essential oils that are released to attract bees, and other pollinators), to ward off predators such as grazing insects or animals, to warn other plants of the approach of predators such as swarms of locusts, for many other reasons. Animals may release pheromones sexual attractants, or as a defence mechanism (for example the skunk).

All these meanings are analysed by the olfactory system which connects directly into the limbic area of the brain and also by the vomer-nasal apparatus; to some extent, we also taste the air both in our mouths and via the taste receptors in our lungs. Humans tend to be extremely visually orientated and do not rely as strongly on their sense of smell like some other species. Smell and odour have strong cultural biases—what we find pleasant or unpleasant will be affected by culture. In the West, we tend to mask our own odours, a way of hiding large amounts of information about ourselves. Our body chemistry and therefore our odour varies depending on our health, our emotional state, our diet and much more besides. For women, their sense of smell varies with their menstrual cycle. Doctors used to use their sense of smell to help with the diagnosis of their patients. We also breathe out other information; CO_2, O_2 and other gaseous substances such as volatile oils from our diet.

The blood returns from our extremities, our feet, to our lungs via the heart to be re-oxygenated; traditionally, this was used as a way of treating the respiratory system, footbaths and foot rubs would be used to treat respiratory infections, excess mucus, spasm in the chest. Garlic or onions would be rubbed on the soles of the feet to help shift mucus and treat infection. Applying essential oils to the feet in rubs or footbaths is also used.

We also have taste receptors in our lungs; although we do not necessarily experience taste in the same way via our lungs it means that footbaths and smoke and smudge are also having an effect on this sense and this is an idea to be explored as we expand our view of how to work with our plant allies.

Our lungs are also one of the main sites of DMT/metatonin production—deep breathing in meditation, the use of incense and smudge may also facilitate this production and our connection to the imaginal realm.

As we breathe out the lungs, provide the form of energy that allows us to express into our external environment by vocalisation. Singing, talking, shouting, chanting, laughing, sighing, even crying are forms of expiration and the way our voice sounds expresses how we feel. If the lungs are out of balance there may be an underlying sadness in our voice (the person who sounds as though they are about to burst into tears all the time), there may be excessive sighing (although this can be a sign of liver imbalance too, or the happy sigh of coming home to our heart); the person who never sings or hums or sticks to a narrow vocal range may be holding all sorts of emotions or may be emotionally detached from the scenario.

When we work with our breath we make it an awareness of our breathing rather than forcing deep breathing; we can relax the diaphragm gently, kindly, in case it is holding emotions and grief (or anger) that we do not feel ready to release, that we have been told is not safe to express, and we have believed it. As the beliefs shift then the ability to release becomes easier.

Air is a form of energy. Breathing in may be perceived as taking in energy, whilst breathing out is releasing energy. Thus, when we are relaxed our breathing cycle is often equal. If we are tense, we will often hold our breath and then release it once the tension has passed. If we are tired or under stimulated, (bored), we may yawn to take in more energy.

When we are tense, we often do not breath properly; most people only breath into the top third of the lungs. Shallow breathing patterns often become habitual in childhood since such patterns can help to cut off feelings and this is what a child will do if the world and the feelings it elicits do not feel safe or are too painful and there is no-one to share that pain with. This means that the rest of the lungs do not get fresh air into them; they are filled with stale air and receive no information. Breathing also helps the circulation, particularly the venous circulation and the circulation of the lymph. Deep breathing facilitates this by expanding the diaphragm down into the abdomen; it also massages the bowel and can help with constipation, or with forms of diarrhoea associated with spasm and tension in the bowel; in TCM, the Lung and Large Intestine meridians are paired together. Deep breathing should not be forced; rather, one moves into an awareness of the breathing patterns and allows the shift to happen to a more healthy one by moving into the parasympathetic or heart space.

There is an intimate relationship between the lungs and the bowel (they are connected by the vagus nerve). If the bowel wall is damaged (irritated or inflamed) it can predispose to asthma and other respiratory conditions. If the lungs are excessively phlegmy this can cause more mucus to be secreted in the bowel; postnasal drips and the swallowing of phlegm can cause a disruption to the digestion, and there are many wise plant healers that work on both at the same time such as *Inula helenium*, *Foeniculum vulgare*, *Marrubium vulgaris*. There can also be effects in the skin; as has been remarked before all the tissues lining the internal organs come from the same embryological tissue. The lungs draw in the oxygen that enables the cellular combustion of the fuel source (glucose, creatinine, glycogen, fat etc.). If we are not drawing in sufficient oxygen, the fire cannot burn brightly. Think of what happens if you put a night light into a closed jar—after a while it will extinguish due to the lack of oxygen. If the tissues do not receive sufficient oxygen, then they start to die.

The upper respiratory tract is lined with hairs and ciliae to trap any particles that are breathed in with the air. Many of the plants that are used to treat respiratory problems are covered in fine white hairs or down—plants such as coltsfoot, mullein, lungwort, elecampane, white horehound. Our respiratory system secretes mucus in order or lubricate and to protect. Problems arise if there is excess secretion, or the secretions become too thick, or if pathogens start to breed in the mucus. Problems can also arise if there is under-secretion of mucus since the respiratory system does not like excess dryness.

If there is an imbalance in the lungs the voice often sounds sad, the skin may appear very white or grey. The breathing may be shallow or laboured.

The upper respiratory system includes the nose which draws in the air, filters and warms it before it goes to the lungs. The nose also contains the olfactory bulb and vomer-nasal organ which read or sense chemical information from the air. The sinuses are an important part of the upper respiratory tract responding to changes in pressure and many other things, and sometimes these can become blocked with uncried tears which may drip down the back of the throat in a postnasal drip or become sensitive to substances contained in the ear. The ears listen to the sound information contained in the air; all these parts form the upper respiratory system. Colds and flus can help to shift unresolved emotions or maybe the body creating a time to slow down and detoxify physically and emotionally. Asthma can be linked to the kidneys (fear), often triggered by a specific trauma and tends to be more stress-related. Or it can be from the lungs as a result of unresolved grief and a tendency to be sensitive.

Part of the human condition is to feel the pain of the world, the more we open into our heart energy, the more we hone our sensory acuity and engage with the conversation of the Universe the more pain we sense; the more we laugh and smile, the more pain we feel. The more we laugh, the more we are able to cope with pain. When we experience change and loss, when we see the wounds around us and within ourselves of course we feel pain, of course we need to mourn. Emotions are not played one at a time; we may feel grief and joy at the same time. When we experience fear, it may move us into anger. In a culture of sanitised emotionality, we feel that emoting is not acceptable and therefore we need to feel less, we need to disengage from the process of living. We are given many aids to accomplish this—television, computer games, cutting off from the rest of the natural world, reducing face-to-face human contact. More and more of our interactions are with computers and machines; the left brain prefers synthetic reality. The right hemisphere, the one connected with the intelligence of the living world is more prone to grieving. Grief is a normal, natural part of our emotional repertoire.

The lungs allow us to feel and express healthy grieving. Grief has many negative connotations in our culture. But we have much to grieve in our lives—each transition has an element of loss, and we need to acknowledge this rather than doing the stiff upper lip, the 'coping well'. Coping well really means allowing those feelings to surface and flow out, from our eyes with floods of tears, from our noses in streams of snot, from our throats as wailing, screams or howls of pure emotion. True grieving takes time and is made up of many stages and may involve the experiencing of a full range of emotions, some of which we may find challenging. If we find some aspects difficult, we need to shine a light on them, bring them forward, rather than run from them: there may be a numbness and difficulty in accepting the loss, a denial that it has happened or has any significance. There may be joy and relief that the person or situation is no longer there; there may be fear around how the change will affect our situation or our ability to function in our situation. There may be anger towards the person who has died, the people we feel are to blame for the loss, ourselves. There may be feelings of guilt about how we dealt with the process of loss, with the processes of severance. There is a lot to deal with and to truly grief is to enter into all the stages and accept them; to see all the parts of the process, including the shadow parts; to fully engage in the process, give ourselves the space to engage with our feelings.

It is generally accepted that it takes 2 years to process a bereavement—and then we will be surprised by the process re-emerging at any time later in our lives.

Knowing that small losses are not to be laughed at—for each of us, different experiences have different emotional significances attached to them. For one person what is a trivial matter to others can be highly emotionally-charged and this needs to be honoured. Sometimes, the more unresolved issues there are around a loss, the more grief and pain is experienced. Sometimes if a loss happens when other losses have not been processed, it can be overwhelming.

Tears

There are three types of tears—basal tears are the tears that continually bathe and moisturise the eye and help to keep it free from infection, irritant tears are those from irritation of the eye by cold or other stimuli. The third type are emotional tears which have a higher protein content since they contain hormones associated with emotions; it would appear that women are more disposed to releasing excess hormones via their tears: they cry four times more often. One of the main hormones released in the tears is prolactin which is present in higher levels in women's bodies which may be one of the reasons women cry more. However, it seems that men release more of their excess hormones by sweating and urinating. Also, it is possible that men in other cultures cry more freely due to it being more accepted during nurture.

The lung time of year is late autumn or early winter. In the medicine wheel cycle, it is aligned to the north, ancestors, the element of Earth and growth. It ties in with Samhain in the Celtic calendar, Halloween or the Day of the Dead (Ancestors) in the Mexican calendar. It is the time in all of our cycles that comes after the emergence of spring, the growth and hard work of summer, the harvesting of autumn. It is the time when we mourn for what might have been, the things we wish we had done and know we never will (but also recognising the things we have not done and that we will do and those that we are glad we did not do!), and the things we wish we had done differently: a time of releasing. As with the breath cycle inspiration and expiration and then a pause. We descend back into the underworld to prepare the soil, plant the seeds, relax, repair, restore or compost if that is where we are in the cycle.

From this time of descending we move through into the element of water. Water is in the North on the medicine wheel; it is the place of the cave, the bear of hibernating and understanding and is associated with the colour black which we now associate with mourning. Black is also associated with shapeshifting—as we understand more, we shift.

Grief rituals

As we have already mentioned grieving is not just about mourning the death of people we love; grieving can be associated with all sorts of life events.

It is important to remember and honour our losses, the people, places and so forth, that are gone; this helps us to grieve. We may need to repeat this process as we move through the spirals of our lives.

Rituals help us acknowledge and mourn loss and also symbolise what we wish to keep in our hearts, and what we cherish; they can help us to commemorate. There are conventional grief rituals such as funerals and memorial services, anniversary masses. However, it can also be helpful to create our own special rituals. In Mexico, when they celebrate the Day of the Dead, they set up altars to their departed friends and ancestors, cook a special meal and put offerings of food on the altars; they may also spend time sitting at the altar speaking with those who have passed on and then as the living share food together; they tell stories of those who have died, or places they have moved on from, or their early lives. Samhain would traditionally have had a similar theme to it: a day when we gather to feast and remember our ancestors at the time of year when we would also mourn those events that did not go well that year.

Grief rituals may be in the form of a memorial meal with a place set for the missing person where people share stories and memories of the person. Groups of immigrants would often traditionally have a day where they would gather to share traditional food and stories to remind them of their homeland. Setting up an altar can be helpful, a space with photographs, maybe flowers or other objects that remind you of the person, the place or the event one is grieving. Or just plan a time for a ceremony. Set a time and make a space; select some music, a poem, some inspirational writing of your own or someone else that you can use to open and close the ceremony. Then decide what else you would like to have in the ceremony, maybe planting a tree or other plant as a remembrance. Because the ceremony is about releasing grief or about grieving allow the emotions to flow. If you need to speak out words, to cry or even scream them, do that. If you need a pile of pillows to pummel to release anger, then make sure that you have some there. A grief ritual may be a solitary event, or you may decide to share it with friends and family. If you have set up a memorial, keep it in place as long as you need it. When you feel your grief is subsiding, you may decide that you need to dismantle your shrine in which case give the same care and attention to do this as you did to making it.

Grief is the natural emotional processing of change and loss. Happiness is not mutually exclusive to grief and happiness is something that comes from within; it is about our relationship with ourself. Maladoma Somé tells how at the funerals in his native village everyone is expected to cry. A funeral is seen as a ritual to mark the death of the person who has just died; it is also seen as an opportunity for the village, for the community, to mourn its little loses as a whole and for people to mourn anything else that they have not mourned sufficiently for.

The story of ivy

I grew up in a medical family—my dad was a doctor, and my mum was a nurse. I was fascinated by plants and their medicinal powers from an early age, and some of the first plants I grew were herbs: I got one of those mixed packs of seeds when I was about 8 and patiently tended the seedlings. When I was 11, I bought my first herbal book—*The Herb Book* by John Lust, followed by a book called *Herbs* with beautiful watercolour illustrations that I used to eat with my eyes. I remember reading *The Armourer's House* by Rosemary Sutcliffe, and I so wanted to be the woman with the herb garden when I grew up. Instead, I went to college and studied Plant Science and Horticulture and worked as a research scientist for 5 years. And then I went to study to be a medical herbalist; well, that's the abridged version, it took me a long time to get qualified as a medical herbalist. And then I was a little confused; there was something missing.

One day I read one of those books that are soul-affirming. When I found out that the author was coming to teach in the UK, I scraped up the money to fly over and hived off to stay with my parents for a weekend to go to the course. And the first day the teacher said that those students who were botanists (aka plant scientists) would find the work very hard—too much head stuff about plants—I was sad. Then he said that any medical herbalists would also find it very difficult—too much head stuff, too many preconceptions about plants. My heart sank doubly at this point; I understood what he meant. So, when we were sent out to sit with a plant, I was determined to find one I knew very little about, to do the exercise well, but I felt that I was possibly the subject of a double whammy. So I walked through the gardens, and my inner botanist ran a commentary of Latin names, crowing with delight at her knowledge, accompanied by my inner medical herbalist eager to put forward her knowledge of constituents, actions and book-learned therapeutics; my inner child and infant were both a little sad, and frustrated—they liked the game they were supposed to be playing, it sounded fun, and they did not like the others spoiling it. I walked past a patch of ivy which drew my attention, but of course I walked past it. I walked in a circle and found myself back with the ivy. It drew me close, and I sat by it and asked it to talk to me if that would be ok; I knew that my inner ears might have some trouble hearing over those authoritative voices, but I would try my best—I wanted to hear her story.

Well, a miracle happened and happened so quickly my heart was bursting. As I looked at the ivy growing over the ground, I saw that the leaves looked like the alveoli in the lungs, spread out to absorb as much oxygen and sunlight as possible in the dark shade where it grew. Precisely ordered leaves, clear black smoke. My inner herbalist piped up with the fact she thought she had read something about ivy and respiratory disease; I told her to play the game properly. The ivy became a woman in a dark green dress; she told me that she draws the old, ancient deep dark grief out of the lung; our own and that passed down from our ancestors, she is kind and clears darkness.

The stems were thin and green/brown in colour. The older leaves were eaten, the young leaves were bright green, spreading, very strong; when my inner child touched it, it entwined on her arms, and she started absorbing green from it. My infant turned towards it, smelling its medicine, and the plant formed a crib to cradle her safely; clearing dark thought patterns. My child said it is like breathing lungs it looks like alveoli; the lady clears out black energy and pain.

I was so excited when we were called back to the classroom.

No-one else would speak up with their experiences so I started to tell my story with great excitement, how I thought I would not be able to communicate with the plants because of my double whammy. The story bubbled up and then all of a sudden I was sobbing, sobbing from beneath the soles of my feet and saying 'I'm sorry'. That was the first time I experienced that gestaltian communication of emotion from a plant, a real demonstration of the kind of energy that ivy shifts, the plants really did give a deep first lesson. Green heart-shaped leaves, as the lungs clear from grief the heart lightens. And the resilience of ivy, a plant that just keeps coming back when it is hacked back.

Examples of herbs for the respiratory system

Achillea, Allium, Althea, Amoracia, Angelica archangelica, Asclepias, Boswellia, Castanea, Cedrus, Cetraria, Chondrus, Citrus sp., Commiphora, Cupressus, Drosera, Eucalyptus, Euphorbia, Euphrasia, Foeniculum, Glechoma, Grindelia, Hordeum, Hyssop, Ilex, Inula, Lactuca, Lavandula, Linum, Lobelia, Lonicera, Malus, Marrubium, Matricaria recutita, Melaleuca sp., Mentha x piperita, Morus, Myrtus, Ocimum, Origanum, Papaver, Picea, Pinus, Plantago, Primula, Prunus, Pulmonaria, Ravensara, Rosmarinus,

Salvia, Sambucus, Saponaria, Schisandra, Styrax, Thymus, Tilia, Trifolium, Tussilago, Ulmus, Valeriana, Verbascum, Viola sp., Zingiber.

Respiratory spasmolytics

Grindelia, Euphorbia, Drosera rotundifolia, Inula helenium, Glycyrrhiza glabra, Lobelia inflata, Valeriana.

Warming

Thymus vulgaris, Cinnamomum verum, Zingiber officinale, Astragalus membranaceus, Ocimum sanctum.

Expectorants

Inula, Thymus, Foeniculum vulgare, Pimpinella anisum, Marrubium Lobelia inflata, Glycyrrhiza, Grindelia.

Antitussives

Prunus serotina (particularly good in tracheitis), *Glycyrrhiza, Bupleurum.* For dry coughs use demulcents also—*Althea officinalis, Hordeum vulgare, Plantago, Pulmonaria officinalis.*

Antiseptic

Inula, Thymus, Allium.

Diaphoretics

Achillea, Asclepias, Melissa officinalis, Mentha x piperita, Sambucus nigra flos, Tanacetum parthenium, Tilia.

Anti-catarrhal

Verbascum thapsus, Plantago lanceolata.

Mucolytic

Allium sativum, Amoracia rusticana. Inhalations of essential oils (eucalyptus, peppermint, rosemary).

Immune enhancing

Astragalus, Echinacea angustifolia, Sambucus nigra fructus.

Anti-inflammatories

Glycyrrhiza, Bupleurum, Rehmannia. Omega 3 rich oils such as linseed, walnut and oily fish.

CHAPTER TEN

The upper cauldron

The neuroendocrine system

The Upper Cauldron or Coire Sois is the cauldron of Wisdom, Knowledge or Inspiration, connected to spirit and is located in the centre of the head around the third eye. For many people, this cauldron is upside down unless they have done the emotional work of filling the second cauldron. Once this is done, we can turn this cauldron upright and start to fill it. We have a natural cycle of development, and we have to proceed through the different stages; we will explore this more when we look at the cycle of maturation in the next chapter.

Although our mental and spiritual faculties are spread through our being, as are our physical and emotional, it is generally agreed that in order to be healthy, well-grounded and embodied we first fill our lower cauldron, then our middle and finally our upper one. So much of 'spirituality' these days focuses on the upper to the detriment of the other two, causing problems and pathologies in our culture. Or perhaps this is a symptom of the same pathology that caused the separation from the land. The one that whispered spirit is separate and the universe has no soul is now whispering to neglect and reject our bodies in favour of spirit, mentation and psyche ... that way lies madness, literally. And we

183

are now seeing raised incidences of anxiety, depression, complex trauma and other conditions as a result. Sadly, people are seeking solutions that worsen the problem rather than heal it.

The Three Cauldrons are a valuable concept and description. However, our sentience, psyche and spirituality is disseminated throughout our being and in constant conversation with the spirit and vitality of the rest of the Universe. Our mind is our whole being and also influenced by the sentience of our microbiomes and the flow of conversation. The neuroendocrine complex is a whole-body system without hierarchy, but lots of feedback loops, spiralling cycles and flows of energy.

The neuroendocrine system

Our brains and nervous system are not a hierarchy but a community reaching decisions by consensus with the appropriate leader for the task at hand who is essentially a servant of the community; dynamic balance when functioning well. Dominance of the Hypothalamus-Pituitary-Adrenal-Sympathetic axis is not the natural mode of being; the parasympathetic, Cordial-Relax-Restore-Repair axis is the mode we would naturally spend more time in; like all animals we are in better health when we are predominantly in the cordial axis, in the heart energy with our bodies entraining to this energy.

In orthodox anatomy and physiology the nervous system is described as a communication system, doing the work of detecting and responding to changes inside and outside the body; nervous tissue is described as being excitable; stimulation of the nervous system evokes immediate responses to changes, whilst the endocrine system tends to be slower and more long-lasting. There has also been the view that we can objectively see reality without our own individual view affecting it.

For several hundred years, the neocortex has been seen as the dominator of the system with our head-brain ruling the rest of the body and neurotransmitters being produced solely within the central parts of the nervous system. However, neurotransmitters are produced in many sites throughout the body; for example, serotonin is produced in the body, the pineal gland and the gut-brain; melatonin is produced in the pineal gland, lungs and thyroid; dopamine is produced in the neurones (nerve cells) and in the adrenals. Neurotransmitters and neuro-peptides are produced in sites throughout the body, and some molecules act as both neuropeptides and hormones. Neuropeptides and neurotransmitters are both used for communication within the nervous system, often working together. Some neurotransmitters are excitatory (glutamate, hence the undesirable effects of monosodium glutamate for many people) and others are inhibitory (GABA, gamma-aminobutyric acid); others such as acetylcholine may be either excitatory or inhibitory, depending on the receptor they are stimulating. Some neurotransmitters are not exciting or inhibiting per se; rather they simply activate a particular metabolic pathway; this rather alters the view that the nervous system is purely a quick response system. We also need to remember the emerging science of psychoneuroimmunoendocrinology (PNIE) which helps to elucidate the interconnectedness of all the systems in our being and how they affect each other; science has begun to recognise that we are complex beings, not machines. The fact that many hormones act as neurotransmitters and vice versa means that the concept of the neuroendocrine system is gaining credibility once more; it does make more sense since these two systems really do work in tandem.

We have already explored the idea that our heart is actually our emotional brain which is in a continuous conversation with our head-brains; in embryological development, the heart develops before the brain and will entrain the neocortex, our emotional intelligence develops before our analytical processing. We have also explored the skin as a sensory brain and the enteric nervous system and made a quick mention of the sacral plexus, which we will look at in more depth in a while. In fact, David Abrams puts forward the possibility that our entire body is a brain that is in constant communication with the consciousness of the Earth, our ecosystem and with the Universe.

Some explorations of nervous tissue

Most orthodox texts state that once the brain is fully developed, we do not produce any new neural tissue, but this has been shown to be erroneous. Spending time in Nature, in our natural state enables us to produce new nerve cells (neurogenesis), to repair our brain tissue. And with the right kind of stimulation, we can rewire our neural pathways, make new connections; this is part of the process of decolonising the brains and reclaiming the indigenous soul. As well as spending time in Nature, phytohormones such as kinetin help neural repair so eating plenty of sprouted seeds, fresh young spring shoots and other forage foods high in plant growth hormones repair and regenerate our nervous tissue and other tissues such as the skin. Anthocyanidins found in cherries, bilberries and other purple/red berries also help neurogenesis, and so do herb robert, *Verbena*, rosemary and *Hypericum* amongst others, including lion's mane fungus.

Triune brain theory

This theory of the brain was put forward by Paul McLean. He suggests that the head-brain is three brains in one; the three layers or brains being the reptilian system/R complex, the limbic system and the neocortex. Each layer has a separate function, but they also work together.

The reptilian brain is made up of the brainstem and cerebellum (which controls balance, muscle coordination and muscle tone) and is mainly concerned with physical survival and maintenance of bodily functions such as digestion, reproduction, circulation, breathing and fight-or-flight response to stress. As it is involved with basic survival, it governs survival behaviours in all animals. It also governs how we all establish home territory, reproduce and strive for social dominance. Reptilian brain behaviours are automatic (what we call instinctual), often have a ritualistic nature and are resistant to change.

The limbic system is viewed as the second part of the brain to evolve. It consists of the amygdala which associates events and emotions and is activated in situations that arouse strong emotions (fear, pity, anger, outrage, grief and deep joy). If it is damaged, emotionally-charged memory can be destroyed. The other part of the limbic system is the hippocampus, which converts information into long-term memory and is involved in memory recall. It is believed that the hippocampus decides which memories are stored by attaching an emotional marker to them. The more the specialised neural pathways in the hippocampus are used the more it enhances memory storage (repetition, repetition, repetition) this applies both to repeated experiences and deliberate study. The limbic system is all about emotion and memory, the expression of emotion, the mediation of emotions and our emotional attachments; these feelings of love and protection are made more complex by the linking up of the limbic system and the neocortex. The limbic system links emotions and behaviours and this moderates the reptilian brain's preference for habitual and ritualistic responses to situations. The limbic system is situated close to the hypothalamus (which is at the top of the endocrine cascade, regulates the ANS and the pituitary, is involved in the regulation of emotional and behavioural patterns, regulation of eating and drinking, control of body temperature, regulation of diurnal rhythms and states of consciousness) and thalamus (which is the conduit for sensory input from the skin). It is directly connected to the olfactory apparatus, and so smell can evoke strong emotions and memories. The limbic system also plays a role in basic responses such as hunger, thirst, sleep, sex and bonding needs.

The neocortex, cerebrum or cerebral cortex is what makes language, speech and writing possible. It is also the part of the brain involved in logical and operational thinking and allows us to plan forward. It is divided into various regions. There are two regions, one governing voluntary movement and another that processes sensory input. There are also the two hemispheres which we will explore further on. Around 90% of right-handed people are apparently left hemisphere dominant and 50% of left-handed people. Some people have equal dominance and more fluidity moving from one to the other.

The *Corpus callosum* is the longitudinal fissure that connects the left and right sides of the brain. It helps communication between the two hemispheres and is the largest area of white matter in the brain. It has been claimed that race and gender affect the size of it. However, there is a lot of dispute about whether this is true. It was purported that it was wider in females, which helped inter-hemisphere communication and therefore a woman's intuition. What does appear to be true is that its size and health can be adversely affected by abusive rearing—shouting and hitting. Given the traditional differences in the rearing of male and female children and the emotional repression of the male perhaps this is not a difference of nature but of nurture. The front part of the *Corpus callosum* has been reported to be larger in musicians, left-handers and ambidextrous people. Brain gym exercises are alleged to help improve left/right hemisphere communication, e.g., cross crawling (definitely babies who do not crawl as part of their development can experience problems with hemisphere communication later in life), hydration, belly breathing, visualising the two hemispheres coming together and working together, certain acupressure points.

The left and right hemispheres and their role in brain function and perception

Iain McGilchrist is a neurologist who has done ground-breaking work in this area, and the following is a summary of some of his research and concepts.

Contrary to popularist views both the left and right hemispheres are actually involved in reason and emotion, and in language and visual acuity. They just do it differently.

The brain is connected but divided by the *Corpus callosum*, and the division has become more extreme through evolution. In mammals and birds, this gives rise to a situation where the two hemispheres actually inhibit each other so that our thoughts and actions come from one or the other depending on which is given prescience.

The left side of the brain has a smaller frontal lobe and a broader posterior lobe. The left hemisphere tends towards narrow, sharp focus and specific and precise description using denotive language and clarity; it gives a simplified view. The left hemisphere is also the part of the brain that enables us to know how to manipulate things and relies on tools to manipulate the world. Its worldview is general in nature; it likes boxes and labels and decontextualizes. Its worldview is lifeless, mechanistic and prefers machines and closed system perfection.

The right hemisphere has a larger frontal lobe and a narrower posterior lobe and is more about broad vigilances and a broader worldview; interconnectedness, social community and pair partners, sustained alertness and attention span. The right hemisphere puts things into context, uses metaphor and reads emotional expression and body language. It reads implicit meanings and allows that things might be different from expectations. The right hemisphere deals with the embodied living world rather than the mechanical; it deals with individuals rather than just categories—it removes labels and takes things out of boxes, changing and evolving. It sees incarnate, living beings in the context of a lived world. It is happy with a broad understanding that may never be totally graspable, or never be fully known.

The two frontal lobes actually inhibit each other and also inhibit the immediacy of experience which allows us to be Machiavellian to read others' intentions and therefore plot and plan, but also to move into that slightly distanced place that allows empathy and bonding; the place of non-attachment, the place of non-activation or reactivity. Both hemispheres are involved in imagination and reason, but they do it a bit differently, creating two versions of the world. All the time we are combining them and as we know some people prefer one view to the other.

As a culture, we have become more and more left-dominant over the last few thousand years. This has led to more emptiness, unhappiness and mental illness. We start to believe that the genius is within us rather than listening to the daemons and geniuses, in the wall in Nature, the external muse as Elizabeth Gilbert describes most eloquently in her talk on nurturing creativity.

As Iain McGilchrist said in *The Master and his Emissary*:

The pursuit of freedom has become replaced by a network of small compli-cated rules that cover the surface of human existence; that compress, enervate, extinguish and stupefy. More and more information is available with less and less opportunity to understand it, to be wise. There is a paradoxical relation-ship between adversity and fulfilment; restraint and freedom; knowledge of or information about and wisdom of the whole. The machine model does not work; even rationality is grounded in a leap of intuition, to trust the rational. Rationality demonstrates its' own limits. The left hemisphere dominated world prioritises virtual over real; the importance of the technical, the technique and form rather than the conversation, the communication, the holistic view; bureaucracy flourishes. The picture becomes fragmented, and there is a loss of uniqueness, How becomes subsumed in what. The need to control leads to paranoia that we need to govern and control everything.

The left hemisphere edits out all that does not fit its model or view; it scotomises and controls the media. It is a hall of mirrors that refuses to see anything that may undercut its view and keeps reflecting back itself.

The right hemisphere does not have an analytical voice that constructs such arguments; perhaps it has a voice but does not argue well, it stops to smell the roses and see the sunrise and the night sky and wonder.

We need the left hemisphere with its ability to reason, careful use of language (both sorely absent at present); we need precise focus, but not at the expense, at the exclusion, of the right hemisphere connection to the living world. In short, we need all our brains, and we need them all connected up.

The blood-brain barrier

The blood-brain is maintained by the choroids plexus of the CNS and is what separates the cerebrospinal fluid from the circulating blood. It prevents bacteria and large or hydrophilic molecules from entering the brain but allows in small molecules like CO_2 and O_2. The cells use active transport to allow metabolically important products like glucose through the barriers. Spirochetes can cross into the CSF by tunnelling through the blood vessel walls which explains why diseases like Lyme disease and syphilis can affect the brain. Large neurotoxins cannot cross the blood-brain barrier so only affect the peripheral nerves. So, the blood-brain barrier protects the brain from foreign substances that may injure the brain; from hormones and neurotransmitters and maintains a constant environment for the CNS. The gut-brain has a similar barrier, but the heart-brain does not; it is natural to be open-hearted.

The reticular activating system

The reticular activating system is a bundle of densely packed nerves in the core of the brainstem between the medulla oblongata and the mid-brain. It runs from the top of the spinal cord to the middle of the brain and contains nearly 70% of the brains 200 billion nerve cells. As well as being involved with the circadian rhythm it is thought to be the part of the brain that is affected by many psychotropic drugs and general anaesthetics, as well as by melatonin, and possibly also serotonin and metatonin. As well as allowing consciousness to occur (bilateral damage causes permanent coma) its fibres are vital for controlling respiration, cardiac rhythms and other essential functions. It appears to be the centre of arousal and motivation in the brain of all mammals. However, it also appears to be the filter of information that is allowed to pass through to a conscious level.

We live in a world that bombards us with information in the form of sounds, visual images and much more. The RAS filters information from the sensory organs, but also from the sensory aspects of the peripheral nerves since if we allowed all this through at a conscious level, we would not be able to process the information, so we need to have a system to screen what it is necessary to pay attention to. The RAS only allows in information that is valuable at the present moment or information that alerts us to a danger or threat to be processed at a conscious level. All information that is perceived as normal, as background, passes up the spinal cord for analysis and processing. Exceptional information passes up through the reticular formation or RAS in the brainstem, bypassing the spinal cord completely. There are eight nuclei in the RAS which act as triage stations for the sensory input of the cranial nerves. Once the RAS identifies information as being exceptional and needing a rapid response (due to it being particularly interesting, or particularly threatening) the information is transmitted to other cranial nerves.

- The vagus (which is also part of the autonomic nervous system, connecting to the major organs and governs things like heart rate, breathing rate, motor feed to the vocal cords for yelling and roaring and growling, pupil dilation, diversion of blood from the digestive organs to the muscles, increase of adrenaline production and other aspects of fear, flight and flight response).
- It also feeds to the trigeminal nerve which supplies the pterygoid muscles in the jaw and the temporalis muscles, preparing us to bare our teeth and bite (many people who are under chronic stress have TMJ problems, grind their teeth, or have problems with temporal tension).
- Both these nerves also supply the ear and may have an effect on sharpening our hearing in the face of danger (another symptom of chronic stress is tinnitus).

For each person the information allowed through will differ depending on their interests (for example, one may notice all the models of car on the road, another may notice all the species of birds and plants in the hedgerow as they travel), and their life experience (one person may perceive the waiter in the restaurant as respectful and helpful, whilst another may find him condescending and snobbish). We may even screen out people who threaten our view of reality, literally not notice that they are there (scotomisation is the ability to ignore people and things that challenge our world view too much).

Given that much of our RAS programming happens when we are under the age of 6 (even before birth) it is good to discover that we can deliberately re-programme the RAS with our conscious mind by goal setting, making affirmations, and using visualisation. By setting a particular goal and removing negative thoughts around it, we can make that the reality of our RAS. The RAS will believe whatever programme you feed it; because it does not distinguish between real events and synthetic reality, visualisations will enhance performance, e.g., rehearsing a speech or a race through visualisation will actually improve our ability to carry out that task. If you like, it is the bridge between our conscious and our subconscious. There is also a negative implication of the RAS not differentiating between real events and synthetic reality. It will be affected by all synthetic information unless we inform it that this is fantasy and does not need to be put into the rapid reaction stream, that it can be totally ignored. This means that all the media input we have can be part of the programming of the RAS. So if you spend all your time watching CSI and playing violent games on the computer the world is really scary; if you feed yourself with information from the fear machine that comes through TV, radio, printed media, the internet, then fear becomes an addiction.

Damage to any part of the system can impact on the whole and result in a chronically elevated RAS. This could possibly be mediated by the myofascial system, but also due to the effects that chronic inflammation has on the adrenal glands and on the balance between the HPA and cordial axes. Compression of the vagus nerve (where it passes through the diaphragm) due to muscle strain during birth can give rise to colic and those babies that just do not sleep as well. Prolonged inflammation in any region can also affect the vagus nerve; for example, IBS, fibromyalgia, colitis, chronic cystitis, autoimmune disease, chronic inflammatory disease and hypersensitivity or atopy. Once a branch of the vagus has been in contact with chronic inflammation, it will become sensitised and give a far stronger reaction to stress in other parts of the organism than it would have done otherwise. Equally, inflammation in the gut may trigger the RAS into a stress response. The trigeminal nerve supplies the tonsils and adenoids so prolonged inflammation in these areas may also give an elevated RAS. Also, displacement of the vertebrae by rotation, lateral subluxation, whiplashes or other traumas can put pressure on the sympathetic ganglia and raise the RAS levels. However, once the system accepts these as OK then they no longer need to cause irritation, we can function with them as part of our natural, healthy state; in conditions such a fibromyalgia, chronic fatigue, TMJ, trigeminal neuralgia tinnitus and others, the person's system is not compensating for the irritation or stressor. This means their body is not incorporating them as part of our health.or can tolerate them once external stresses do not exceed a certain limit.

In Victorian times, many women were afflicted with conditions such as neurasthenia, hysteria, 'spleen' and spinal irritation; women in particular seemed to be affected (or labelled). These conditions were felt to have no medical explanation. Neurasthenia was a condition characterised by mental and physical exhaustion, aches and pains, difficulty concentrating and memory loss; hysteria was characterised by muscular aches and pains, backache, frequent urination, vomiting, diarrhoea and violent headaches; spleen imbalance was thought to create black humours and vapours that led to melancholia; spinal irritation was unexplained back pain and was treated by spending years flat on one's back in a health spa. These syndromes have their modern counterparts: chronic fatigue syndrome, with extreme tiredness, musculoskeletal aches and pains, loss of memory and depression which affects a significant number of secondary school children and has become more prevalent as lifestyles become more Westernised. The type of people who are likely to develop this syndrome are high achievers who are attempting to conform to the modern culture where one is expected to achieve at work, at home and often in a field that would not be the first choice for the individual; they take a career path to please their family or social group. Unexplained back pain, similar to spinal irritation affects at least 15% of the population. Migraine affects a large number of women and teenage girls, but also occurs in men and is characterised by photophobia, violent headaches, sometimes vomiting and nausea and even paralysis. Fibromyalgia is characterised by sore muscles and persistent pain, often flitting. Irritable Bowel Syndrome affects 15–20% of the population and is characterised by spasms in the colon, diarrhoea and/or constipation, bloating and intolerance of some foods. Unexplained chest pain affects 20% of the population. Globus syndrome is a sensation of a lump in the throat with no known cause. Dyspepsia affects up to 40% of the population. Candidiasis is characterised by abdominal pain, constipation, diarrhoea, wind, bloating, belching, indigestion, recurrent vaginal candida infection, nasal congestion, sinus problems, bad breath, allergies, chemical sensitivities, rectal itching, muscle aches, fatigue, depression, irritability, headaches, dizziness and difficulty concentrating. Dr Nick Read believes that many of these syndromes are a reaction to modern Western lifestyles. Arthur Kleinman, a medical anthropologist, also feels that conditions such as chronic fatigue syndrome are cultural diseases caused by the drive to high achievement, combined with the isolation in society that means that people who are working long hours often have to combine this with child-rearing or caring for elderly parents, or both; this all leads to a state of complete mental and emotional depletion and a state of exhaustion and despair. It would appear that human beings are social animals with a need for community; as we have seen before, there needs to be a balance between individuality and being part of a collective—not collectivism or individualism but a knowing, a sense of the fact that we are both separate and connected.

Dr Read also makes the point that the reason why many of these syndromes respond better to complementary therapies and psychotherapy is because of the nature of the therapeutic relationship in these areas. The importance of providing a space where the patient can tell their story and know that they are truly being listened too.

The vagus nerve

The vagus nerve was for a while thought of as 'just one of the cranial nerves'. Its very name implies it is a wandering vagabond of a nerve, meandering around the body to nearly everywhere (not the adrenals though). It is one of the cranial nerves, but it is also a huge part of the balance between the sympathetic and parasympathetic pathways of our autonomic nervous system. The nerve starts in the brainstem, just behind the ears and travels in multiple branches that diverge from two thick stems rooted in the cerebellum and brainstem, down each side of the neck across the chest and down into the lowest reaches of the abdomen. It connects from the brain to the lungs, the heart, the spleen the guts, the kidneys and the reproductive organs amongst other places. It also networks with the nerves involved in speech, facial expression, eye contact and much more. It receives stimulation from a lot of these organs, and the information it receives can be very influential on whether we feel relaxed, confident, capable and energetic (toned) or stressed and alarmed. It conveys information from the different centres back to the brain to get a consensual decision. Stress, inflammation, trauma, or tension in any region can cause an overall lack of balance or tone or lead to some quite unusual symptoms that are often dismissed as being hypochondria or psychosomatic, or all in the head. The vagus nerve can produce quite pronounced symptoms without the presence of organic disease process, but these can be extremely debilitating to people. This happens when the parasympathetic activation of the vagus nerve does not kick in to balance out sympathetic response to adrenaline and cortisol by releasing neurotransmitters like acetylcholine and GABA to slow us down. The symptoms of loss of vagal tone can be many and varied and may range from:

- Earache with no physical cause. Or other symptoms in the ears such as tinnitus or itching
- A sensation of tightness or a lump in the throat and difficulty swallowing

- Neck tension
- A sensation of pressure in the chest
- Tachycardia, palpitations, or skipped beats
- Stuttering
- Sensations of breathlessness
- Tingling and numbness or Raynaud's type symptoms in the hands and/or feet
- Epigastric pain, stomach cramps or butterflies in the stomach
- Strange flitting pains in the intestines
- Faintness, dizziness, light-headedness
- Nausea
- Sensations of being extremely hot or cold accompanied by sweating
- Fuzzy thoughts, a slight inability to form words
- Weakness
- Visual disturbances such as lights seem too bright, fuzzy or tunnel vision or black spots in the vision
- Nervousness
- Shaking
- Frequent urination
- A desire for copious amounts of cold water
- And others too many to mention

The symptoms of vagal imbalance can be acute or chronic, depending on how healthy the vagus nerve is and how well it has retained its ability to return to tone. Chronic conditions can severely affect vagus tone.

Good vagal tone is when the parasympathetic part of the vagus nerve is able to kick in under pressure so that one can relax into dealing with a situation. However, many people today have gone beyond the point of healthy stress into a less coping place; this particularly true amongst many young people. Symptoms can also arise after a period of illness or extreme physical stress or trauma such as a car crash or fall. Extreme or prolonged emotional stress can also cause an imbalance. For example, a young woman who came to me (the doctors had told her there was nothing wrong). She would get severe stomach cramps, craved large quantities of cold water and suffered painful spasms during and after sexual intercourse. She was extremely stressed about college studies and the environment in which she was studying.

There are various techniques that can help to engage good vagal tone such as visualisation; cold water splashed on the face; using neuroplasticity; re-wiring, physical exercise, avoiding anxious people and much more besides.

The endocrine system

In conventional anatomy and physiology texts, the endocrine system is described as consisting of the seven endocrine glands which secreted hormones into the blood to alter the physiology of distant organs and tissues. Many people have drawn connections between these and the Chakra system of Ayurvedic philosophy and others have drawn connections between the Chakras and the Cauldrons. There is a connection between the endocrine glands and the Chakras energy centres that can be a helpful way to explore our hormones since the Chakras are not seen as a hierarchy but as a system of energetic centres that all need to be in balance for the being to be well.

There is no hierarchy in the endocrine system; as we have seen, most of the organs produce hormones, and the hormonal system is maybe a better concept to embrace. The pituitary has been described as the master gland at the top of the hierarchy, in command. However, as we have seen with the triune brain it is not in charge, rather they analyse information, make decisions, send out messages, provide for the community in service. They clear communication, maintain consciousness, bring issues to consciousness.

The endocrine system is another communication system within the body that works alongside the others that we have examined; it is an internal system of communication but also allows communication within the environment. For example, aldosterone is a hormone that is produced within the system but is also perceived in a pheromonal way by other organisms. An experiment was conducted where isolated aldosterone was sprayed onto a chair in a waiting room; the women coming into the room chose that chair out of preference to sit on, whilst the males avoided it. Another example is the way in which the male hormones produced by boars have the effect of bringing female piglets into puberty earlier and also affect the menstrual cycle of female human pig farmers. Groups of women will often start to menstruate synchronously after a period of time living together. There is a cross over between pheromones and hormones; oestrogen and other hormones will also have an environmental and communal effect. We all know that if someone is experiencing extreme fear, we 'smell' it and it can be extremely infectious. Intense bliss and ecstasy can be the same.

Interestingly, the perception and action of certain hormones, their actual physiological and psychological effects can be different according to what we expect, our preconceptions and where we are emotionally at a particular time. In one experiment, subjects were injected with adrenaline and told it was a sedative; instead of going into fight-or-flight, they found it calming! The effects of hormonal shifts during the menstrual cycle, during pregnancy and during menopause can differ widely depending on how the woman is in her emotional life. How a man reacts to the lowering of levels of androgens produced during andropause can vary considerably too. Men actually have a cycle of hormone production; it is about 33 days long, so they have what one researcher calls a manstrual cycle with emotion swings but no physical evidence of the changes they are experiencing.

The lower cauldron

Base chakra. The adrenal glands relate to the base chakra, survival fear and courage, and to the ego. Our ego does not need to be killed or excised; it is an innate natural part of ourselves. However, we need to make friends with our ego because it is very good at doing its job of making us fearful when it fears for our survival, and so we need to learn to listen and discuss and then it knows it is valued and will stand out of the way at the times when we need to be empty of ego fear to do our work. Cortisol actually rises when we are in the first stages of falling of love, that blissful state; well, it is quite an inflammatory process, and we do need to open our boundaries and be prepared to deal with wounds. However, similar to the birth process plenty of oxytocin is produced to balance the action of cortisol. In the same way that oxytocin balances the action of adrenaline in the child birthing process. Falling in love can happen with ideas, projects, our work, a place, life, a person, or a piece of art.

Sacral chakra. The gonads (uterus, large bowel, prostate, ovaries, testes). Oestrogen and testosterone; both men and women produce both these substances. Men's oestrogen levels are currently being altered by xeno-oestrogens in the environment. When women move into high-powered, high-stress lifestyles their androgen production rises. Testosterone tends to give the single-minded, approach, the archetypical male mode of operating, left brain, focused activity. Oestrogen gives the ability to multi-task, to nurture, to carry out the archetypical female roles of nourishing and creating. Alteration of the balance can significantly affect behaviours.

In the female, oestrogen is predominantly produced from the gonads until menopause in a monthly cycle; some women continue to produce oestrogen from their ovaries after they stop menstruating and are no longer fertile. It produces the female secondary sexual characteristics of larger breasts and broader hips. It prevents many degenerative diseases such as osteoporosis and heart disease. It helps improve good sleep quality, sensitivity to odours, general sensory acuity and memory. Oestrogen is associated with female sexual behaviour, neuron growth and improved cognition, more stable moods and a sense of wellbeing. Oestrogen is also associated with how women defend themselves. Men produce oestrogen from their adrenals and need some oestrogen to maintain strong bones; men involved in caretaking produce more oestrogen.

Testosterone is produced in the gonads by men and in the adrenals by both sexes. Men produce 10 times more testosterone than women. Testosterone secretion in men depends on gaining a higher place in the social order, attaining leadership positions, becoming the Alpha male. Women who compete in the workplace are likely to produce more testosterone than those who work in the home as carers. Testosterone produces physical characteristics such as body hair, increased muscle bulk, larger bone structure. Emotionally, testosterone creates a sense of separateness, assertiveness, self-confidence, sex drive (rather than affection), aggression, risk-taking, interest in moving objects (cars, planes and the like), and visual-spatial ability. It can also produce anxiety, poor concentration, violent, criminal or psychotic behaviour.

The middle cauldron

Solar plexus (pancreas, liver, spleen, stomach, small intestine). Insulin is one hormone is produced in the pancreas (an organ with Earth energy). Problems arise if insufficient is produced. However, sometimes diabetes is due to the fact that the tissues become resistant to the insulin produced; more of an autoimmune issue. Insulin encourages the storage of sugars whilst glucagon encourages the release of sugars, depending on whether we are preparing for physical activity or resting and restoring and building. Our solar plexus is also the meeting point between the lower and upper chakras; the place where the energy from above reaches down and vice versa. It is the place where we process the information that floods in from the world and where we digest it energetically.

Heart (thymus, heart, breasts). The Heart itself produces several hormones.

Throat (thyroid, lungs, throat, intestines). The thyroid hormones are very much associated with growth, repair and metabolism, metabolic rate; think about the correlation between metabolism and self-expression. There are also the parathyroid glands which are associated with our bone metabolism and balance, perhaps to do with knowing who we truly are and our connection with our ancestors? Also, the heart and thyroid develop from the same tissue embryologically—the thyroid then migrates up to the throat. Think about the link between self-love and self-expression; the throat sings our heart song. Alongside the thyroid (relating to our heart song) are the parathyroid glands which produce hormones that help to maintain healthy bones. So, our heart song and our connection to the ancestors are intrinsically, intimately connected.

The upper cauldron

Third eye (pituitary, eyes, lower head, sinuses). The pituitary is in synergy with the hypothalamus part of the brain, they communicate closely, and the pituitary receives much information from the nervous system this way in order to help it to do its work, but it is often called the master gland due to the fact it regulates growth via growth hormone, the activity of the gonads, the activity of the thyroid, the activity of the adrenals. The posterior gland produces oxytocin and vasopressin, which are thought to play a role in our bonding behaviour with our community as well as the other roles. It is probably not the master but rather a coordinator.

Crown (pineal, brain). The pineal gland is primarily concerned with producing neurotransmitters that also may act in a hormonal way: melatonin, serotonin and metatonin.

Hormonal activity in the body is full of feedback loops, cascades, dances between the chemical messages; the electrical messages and responses to internal and external change; the target tissues and receptors for the hormones, and they balance one another. It is all about homeodynamis—allowing ourselves to adapt our internal environment so that we express ourselves into the external environment.

The endocrine system and the nervous system are closely linked. Actually, it used to be called the neuroendocrine system, and this way of looking at ourselves can give a more rounded, holistic view. Many neurotransmitters have been shown to act like hormones, and some hormones also act as neurotransmitters. In both systems, there is no hierarchy in truth; there is connection and constant communication. The parasympathetic HPA axis is not dominant; it works with the cordial parasympathetic axis; the form of the cross a sacred and central symbol in many cultures.

Neurotransmitters, neuropeptides, hormones and endogenous psychoactives

Neuropeptides are small chain molecules composed of amino acids (like small proteins) that are part of the communication systems between neurons. They have an influence on neural function and activity. They are made and released by the neurons and often work in synergy with neurotransmitters; they are released at the same time. There are specific neuropeptides for each neurotransmitter. Many of them are also hormones, for example, vasopressin, oxytocin, somatostatin. The differentiation between a neuropeptide and a peptide hormone is what cells release them and respond to them. Neuropeptides are secreted from neuronal cells, and signal to neurons whilst peptide hormones are produced and secreted by neuroendocrine cells and travel via the blood to distant tissue to have their effect.

Neurotransmitters are chemicals used by neurons to transmit signals from a neuron to a target cell across a synaptic clef; upon release, they diffuse across the synapse and reach receptors at the other side. Their release is triggered by action potentials (chemical changes in the neuron) and electrical stimuli; there is also a low-level release that is in continuous flow.

Hormones travel through the blood to target tissues at some distance. The action of neurotransmitters is fast whilst the effect of hormones can last from a few seconds to a few days. Hormones regulate.

Often substances function as both neurotransmitters and hormones; this depends on the same criteria as above and includes oxytocin, vasopressin and norepinephrine or noradrenaline. This re-enforces the findings of PNIE, and the complex of the neuroendocrine system is reinstated. Once again, we see that the nervous system and endocrine system are not separate. Furthermore, as we have journeyed through the body, we have discovered that hormones are not just released from the endocrine glands of the HPA axis but also by many other organs including the intestines, the stomach, the heart, kidneys and so on. We have seen how many of the hormones released from these other organs are involved in the parasympathetic rest, restore repair mode.

So, the endocrine system is more properly seen as part of the neuro-endocrine system, and this is seen as having two axes: the HPA axis and the cordial axis.

We have also discovered that we have many brains connected by the vagus nerve. We have explored the head-brain, the heart-brain and the enteric brain to some extent and now will look at the sacral plexus, another brain, and how it is linked via the vagus nerve to the other brains. The sacral plexus is larger and more complex in women due to the fact it has more to coordinate what with periods and childbirth, whilst the head-brain tends to be larger in the male. The sacral plexus does not just co-ordinate reproductive function; it also affects our emotional tone and stores information about our safety. Apparently, it becomes triggered into feeling unsafe if injured by a physical impact such as a fall or car crash or by sexual abuse, but it also becomes alerted by language that is abusive in a sexual context so women who have been verbally abused can display similar trauma reactions to those who have experienced physical, sexual abuse; this may also be true for males, but there is a dearth of information pertaining to the sacral plexus in the male.

What becomes apparent is that the neuroendocrine system is complex and that our mental and spiritual health and awareness is not just centred in the head. A small but interesting observation is that women's head-brains may tend to be smaller than men's, but their sacral brains are larger and vice versa. This may be an adaptation to the different roles of male and female as regards reproduction.

As mentioned earlier for each psychoactive plant constituent our bodies produce an analogous substance, which partly why such substances produce physiological, emotional, mental and spiritual effects. We are co-evolved with plants from the same ancestors, and we share quite a bit of chemistry.

Opiates-endorphins. We produce 20 types of these neurotransmitter polypeptides from the pituitary and hypothalamus.

DMT-metatonin is produced in the pineal gland along with melatonin. And possibly also in the lungs.

Examples of herbs for the nervous system

Trophorestoratives: *Avena, Pulsatilla, Rosa, Rosmarinus, Stachys, Turnera, Verbena.*

Stimulants: *Camellia, Coffea, Cola vera, Angelica, Foeniculum, Pimpinella, Ocimum, Artemisia, Centella, Bacopa, Theobroma.*

Relaxants: *Aloysia, Anthemis nobilis, Asperula, Atropa belladonna, Cananga, Crataegus, Citrus aurantium flos, Datura, Eschscholzia, Humulus, Hyoscyamus, Hypericum, Lactuca virosa, Lavandula, Matricaria, Melissa, Passiflora, Petasites, Piscidia, Primula, Ruta graveolens, Scutellaria, Tilia, Turnera, Valeriana, Viburnum opulus.*

Analgesics: *Hypericum, Mentha x piperita, Valeriana, Passiflora, Melaleuca species, Eugenia, Stachys, Lavandula, Citrus aurantium, Eucalyptus species, Melissa, Cymbopogon species, Matricaria.*

Special senses: *Centaurea cyanus, Euphrasia, Glechoma, Rosmarinus, Vaccinium, Stachys.*

So how does this alter our way of viewing herbs and their nervine actions? What it does show is that herbs can be beneficial nervines by improving heart health, gut health, digestive function, gut flora, vagal tone and probably many other mechanisms that we have yet to understand. So as regards the herbs that we use, what are the potential nervine qualities of herbs and their constituents beyond those we have tended to concentrate on? Well, here are some suggestions:

Cyanogenic glycosides have been shown to balance vagal tone. This can reduce blood pressure, relax the bronchi and the bowel. All of this in turn makes us feel more relaxed and therefore improves mood (or encourages us to take rest and time out when we need it, rather than being driven forward by an excess of adrenal energy). Herbs that contain cyanogenic glycosides include *Prunus serotina* bark and the bark and fruits of other cherry species, *Sambucus nigra* flowers and fruit, (Glennie Kindred has mentioned the value of the flowers for anxiety), *Achillea millefolium.*

Cardiac glycosides improve the tone of the heart, regularity and force of the beat and so forth. When the heart function is healthy, we produce a significant number of neurotransmitters, hormones and other mood enhancing substances from this organ; substances that boost our immune system and make us feel more relaxed. Cardioactive glycosides were originally discovered in foxglove, but most of us are no longer permitted to prescribe that herb. However, they are also found in *Scrophularia nodosa, Cheiranthus, Asclepias, Kalanchoe pinnata, Convallaria majalis* (some of these are still permitted to use this I think).

Glucosolinates are the mustardy substances found in the Brassicaceae for the main part. Their nervine function is via their effect on the enteric nervous system. Small doses stimulate and enhance the immune system; larger doses are emetic. They would appear to have a warming stimulating effect in the guts which will have a reflex arc back to the triune brain, producing a clearing sensation and relieving sluggish moods. They also have a suppressive effect on thyroid function; overactive thyroid is often accompanied by anxiety and episodes would appear to be precipitated in some case by stress and anxiety.

We know that most alkaloid-containing plants have a significant effect on the nervous system, and I am not going to list all the different classes. However, alkamides or alkylamides occur in a range of plants including *Echinacea species, Achillea millefolium, Spilanthes, Amaranthus* and are termed phytocannabinoids. Catechins from *Camellia sinensis* also act on our cannabinoid receptors; our endogenous cannabinoid is anandamide, and *Theobroma coca* contains this substance and also contains substances that slow its break down. This helps us to understand why chocolate and tea have such relaxing effects. It also means that we can expand our view of the therapeutic value of *Echinacea* and *Achillea* for people who are stressed and run down. They not only improve immune function and tissue repair; they help with the stress and fatigue and relax the nervous system which creates positive feedback for oxytocin production and repair. Some work indicates that polyphenols, including anthocyanins, may act on these receptors as well. Also, resveratrol, curcumin, and substances found *in Ruta graveolens, Acmella oleracea, Helichrysum umbraculigerums, Saccharomyces cerevisiae, Rhododendron species, Amorpha, Glycyrrhiza, Radula marginata*, black pepper, kava, maca, black truffles, and flax seeds. It would appear that our extensive endocannabinoid system is an intrinsic part of how we interrelate with plants, or rather how animals and plants interrelate. As one of our graduates commented, it would be mighty strange to have such an extensive system that only reacted to one plant. The ECS is being revealed to play an important role in many areas of health such as appetite, pregnancy, mood, blood pressure, fertility, pancreatic function, liver health; it appears to be spread throughout our tissues and play a role in regulating every physiological system in the body. And apparently, omega 3 oils are really helpful for treating ECS deficiency so plenty of linseed, hemp seed and walnuts.

Bitters have traditionally been used to treat depression. Some of this has been thought to be due to the constituents having effects on the head-brain; for example, the xanthones in *Gentiana lutea* are considered to have a similar structure to MAOI drugs. Others felt it was due to clearing the liver, or because of the energetic quality that bitters have of opening the heart; these are all true. However, bitters also have a significant effect on the gut-brain, and when the gut-brain feels happy, the head-brain is more likely to. So, bitters probably work on all the brains.

Bitters have a wonderful range of actions on vagal tone since they open the heart and circulation, work on the gut-brain and clear the liver and gall bladder amongst other things. There are several classes of bitters and the ones chosen depend on several factors, not least whether the person needs warming (the type who goes cold when vagal tone is not good), cooling (the type who gets hot and sweaty when vagal tone is challenged), or needs balancing (they get temperature fluctuations when vagal tone is compromised).

Bitters are invaluable for balancing vagal tone since they work on the heart, the gut-brain, the liver and on the nervous system. There are several classes of bitters and the bitter chosen for a particular individual depends on their particular condition.

Warming bitters are valuable for those who find that they become cold, with low blood pressure and pallor. These include *Inula helenium*, *Angelica archangelica*, *Citrus aurantium flos*, *Rosmarinus officinalis*.

Cooling bitters are more suitable for those who experience flushing, heat and elevated blood pressure and include *Arctium lappa*, *Verbena officinalis*, *Gentiana lutea*, *Erythrea centaurea*, *Cyanara scolymus*.

Balancing bitters normalise the temperature and are good for those who experience alternating heat and cold; examples are *Matricaria recutita* and possible *Stachys betonica*. Stachys does a lovely visual description of the vagus nerve with its pink flowers held on rather wiggly stems reaching down to firmly anchored roots and leaves reminiscent of the pancreas.

Spasmolytics such as *Mentha x piperita*, *Valeriana officinalis* and *Viburnum species* relax any tension in the body and the smooth muscle and part of their ability to improve cognitive function and learning may well be via relaxation of the gut-brain.

Essential oils are well known to be valuable nervine constituents working on the limbic system in the head-brain but probably affect many other parts of the nervous system as well, especially the enteric nervous system when herbs containing these substances are ingested. A thorough exploration of this would take pages or books, but it is fun to start exploring them:

Ones with a volatile oil rich in esters have a calming effect on the central nervous system and induce better parasympathetic tone, releasing stress, shock and tension in the system. These include *Lavandula* species, *Cananga odorata*, *Pelargonium asperum*, *Anthemis nobilis*, *Citrus reticulata*, *Citrus aurantium flos*. *Citrus aurantium flos* is traditionally used in Lebanon as a 'rescue remedy' for clearing shock and trauma. It contains a volatile oil rich in esters which reset the CNS releasing trauma, but it is also a gently warming bitter and seems to help balance the pancreas.

Plants with volatile oil rich in phenyl methyl ethers include *Foeniculum vulgare*, *Angelica archangelica*, *Pimpinella anisum*, *Ocimum basilicum* and *Ocimum sanctum*. These are rather more warming and stimulating but will improve both sympathetic and parasympathetic tone in small to moderate doses. Large doses can induce too much sympathetic stimulation.

Plants rich in monoterpenes include *Pinus sylvestris*, *Boswellia serrulata*, *Citrus limomum*, *Piper nigrum*, *Picea* species. These are particularly good at improving vagal tone in the respiratory area although they will also work on other areas. The pines and spruce are particularly valuable for relaxing and expanding the lungs but also help balance the neuroendocrine complex (acting on the HPA axis) and thereby improve vagal tone.

Plants containing aldehyde rich volatile oils include *Melissa officinalis*, *Alyosia triphyllata*, *Cymbogon citratus*. These exhibit different actions depending on the dose. Smaller doses are relaxing and improve vagal tone, lowering high blood pressure and relieving digestive spasm. However, higher doses can become over stimulating and irritating.

Plants rich in ketones can be wonderful. We have to be a little cautious with some of them since used for too long or in too high a dose some ketones become neurotoxic and can have the reverse effect to the desired one, so they are often used in low dose or for a minimum of about three weeks then a break is taken. Herbs rich in these constituents include Hyssop (used to treat epilepsy), rosemary, sage, mugwort, wormwood and thuja (all rich in thujone), fennel, peppermint and immortelle (*Helichrysum italicum* whose ketones are non-toxic). Jasmine flowers also contain non-toxic ketones. These plants all have a marked effect on parasympathetic tone.

There are many other examples of other herbs containing volatile oils and oils that are rich in other constituents, but this gives some idea of how valuable herbs of this type (and the essential oils extracted from them) are for improving vagal tone.

Mucilage rich herbs have several values; they act as prebiotics which encourages a healthy gut flora, and our gut flora balance has been shown to be really important for mood and cognitive function. They also reduce inflammation in the gut which reduces stress responses and cortisol levels (this works both ways as high cortisol can increase gut inflammation).

Tannins astringe the gut wall which can help to reduce inflammation and leaky gut effects on the immune system, adrenal hormone balance and other systems.

Probiotics (these include plant-based ones such as cider vinegar, sauerkraut, kimchi, kvass, water kefir, miso and other fermented foods) have been shown to help with mood and memory. They have been shown to be effective for depression, anxiety, ADD, dementia. Basically, a healthy gut flora has benefits for our mood and memory.

Calcium and magnesium rich herbs will definitely work on most parts of the nervous system due to the importance of calcium in neural transmission. They are especially valuable for healthy function of the heart-brain.

Essential fatty acids, especially omega 3 oils, have been shown to improve vagal tone. So, the traditional view of walnuts being good for the brain is very accurate; they are probably good for the entire nervous system via the vagus nerve.

These are just a few sound bites but, by exploring further, we can move to a more holistic view of what the plants' medicine is and so see that we do not need to prescribe one herb for the nerves and another for each physical symptom—they all work on all levels. They always knew that, and some of our elders knew that too, we just have to learn some more and some more depth about our green allies.

Valeriana officinalis has the happy ability to block our response to the excitatory neurotransmitters, calming us whilst improving our concentration and physical capacity. It is quite a heating remedy, so it is not so suited for those with a lot of trapped heat.

Geranium robertianum balances blood sugars, balances blood pressure, encourages neurogenesis which only occurs when the being feels safe and relaxed in the oxytocin zone of rest, repair, regenerate, resolve.

Capsicum can help due to its 'the slap in the face' effect. A wee shock that helps jolt the vagus nerve back into tone.

Other groups of herbs can help due to the fact they reduce stress in the system or improve resilience to stress; the adaptogens or nutritive tonics of which there are many examples in our indigenous and naturalised flora such as *Sambucus nigra fructus, Arctium lappa, Taraxacum officinale, Inula helenium, Salvia officinalis, Rosmarinus officinalis, Plantago major/lanceolata.*

Herbs that are calming nervines can help by reducing sympathetic stimulation and improving parasympathetic tone thus rebalancing and include *Scutellaria lateriflora* and *Verbena officinalis*, along with *Melissa officinalis* and many others.

The heart is the largest and most powerful electromagnetic resonator and centre of neural tissue in the body. As such the heart is the organ that is most able to balance vagal tone. If the heart is happy, then this has a wonderful effect on vagal tone, so heart herbs such as *Leonorus cardiaca, Passiflora incarnata, Crataegus, Tilia, Theobroma, Rosa, Foeniculum vulgare, Melissa officinalis* and *Rosmarinus officinalis* are excellent ones to consider.

Several of our endogenous chemicals are involved in improving vagal tone and allowing us to move through trauma and stress, releasing the trauma of the events so that although we remember the event we do not continually revisit the pain of this. A classic example is the way our hormones assist in childbirth (one of the hardest labour of love) where we release a balance of adrenaline and oxytocin to allow the work to be done (the stressful event to be dealt with), but we also release large amounts of endorphins. Afterwards, we produce a substance called anandamide which is our endogenous cannabinoid—cocoa contains anandamide, proanthocyanidins fit into the cannabinoid receptors, and blueberry has been suggested as a treatment for PTSD (*Vaccinium myrtillus* does similar work as does elderberry, hawthorn, rosehip and sour cherries). *Echinacea* alkamides also fit into these receptors, and this herb has been shown to help treat fatigue and burnout. *Capsicum* constituents also fit into these receptors, possibly part of this herb's slap in the face to re-centre effect. The appropriate stimulation of these receptors can help with vagal tone and rebalancing for sure.

Any herb that stimulates or improves gut tone will help with vagal tone since if the gut-brain is not happy we find it hard to relax and concentrate, to learn and perform well—contrary to present techniques in schooling in many places we actually learn better in community and cooperation rather than being encouraged to compete against others or ourselves or being forced into stressful tests and short fire questions which elicits answers from the adrenalized fear flight sympathetic system or causes a freeze. Having said that with good vagal tone the parasympathetic balances this to move towards fun solutions and engagement of creativity. This is not often welcomed in classrooms but is a great bonus in the real world especially with the challenges we face at present. Plants such as mustard, horseradish and wasabi, wild rocket all help with gastrointestinal tone and clear the sinuses. *Capsella bursa-pastoris* is helpful for improving womb tone and reducing bleeding (along with *Geranium robertianum*, *Mentha species* and *Vaccinium myrtillus*). Vagal tone is really important for womb health, and excess bleeding can be a good indication of stress. It is interesting though anyhow. Some of all these remedies effect on the womb may be mediated by their effect of mucous membranes and capillary tone, but these are strongly affected by the balance of the vagus nerve.

In one way, all this information is irrelevant, but since the importance of the vagus nerve has been revealed once again and explains various symptoms most excellently it is valuable to engage with our allies to see what they have to say about how they work on this level.

It has been discovered that we have taste and smell receptors throughout our bodies and scientists are wondering why. Could it be that when we get a taste in our mouth, it is not just the liver that has a reflex action. What if the sour receptors in the spine respond to this taste via the vagus nerve, the bitter receptors in the heart and sinuses respond via this route (rose and cocoa for the heart and yarrow for the sinuses), the sweet receptors in the kidney/adrenal complex respond to sweet taste explain part of the action of *Codonoposis* and liquorice and a cup of warm, sweet milk tea if shocked or surprised. This is all supposition and hypothesis, but that is where good explorations start from.

In truth, the vagus nerve is intimately involved in garnering information from both our internal and external environments; it senses taste, smell, touch, sound, sight, electromagnetic information and all our sensory input. When it is toned and balanced it becomes less reactive, more able to just sense and discern what is helpful and what is not and to elicit reactions in line with that information (such as vomiting if too much is taken) and then go back to a calm state.

Examples of Herbs for the Endocrine system

Borago officinalis, Cyanara scolymus, Eleutherococcus senticosus, Fucus vesiculosis, Galega, Glycyrrhiza glabra, Rosmarinus officinalis, Serenoa serrulata, Schisandra, Stachys officinalis, Vitex, Withania, Asparagus racemosus.

CHAPTER ELEVEN

The cycles of life

There are two events that are certain in life—our birth and our death.

When we are born, we have the choice of what we do with our one wild and precious life, as Mary Oliver says in her poem 'The Summer Day'.

The cycle of conception, birth, life, death, rebirth is there throughout the Universe.

Reproduction

Our cells are reproducing continually; we completely replace our cells every 7 years, which ties into some theories of the cycles within our lifetime. Physically you are no longer the person you were 7 years ago, except our body memory means that we are (paradoxically); and that is the same spiritually, mentally and emotionally too, hopefully. At the same time, we have our core truth, our authentic self that we adhere to, but it can evolve and be expressed in various ways. Gaia, the natural world of which we are a part, is in a continuous process of reproduction; we notice it especially as we enter the spring, but the process is continuous around the globe with periods of full growth and quiescent periods in the more temperate zone. These cycles are mythologised in stories such as Persephone going into the underworld for several months of the year to spend time with Hades, or the precursor to this of the descent of Inanna to meet her shadow self. More accurately we all need to travel down into the underworld to meet our shadow self both masculine and feminine; Daverick Leggett says in his book *Recipes for Self-Healing* when it is time to do this it is best to take a source of light and a good sense of humour (humour is essential for driving away the shadows and demons). We need to bring the shadowy parts of ourselves to consciousness, learn to dialogue well with them and then emerge after the winter to ascend again. We only need to look at the web of Nature to see Gaia's cycles happening, and we are part of this.

The world is continually reproducing its dream. Within the human species there is also a continuous process of reproduction of thoughts and culture; we are involved in reproducing the human dream and evolving to be in alignment with the world dream; we are part of the world's endeavours to dream itself to health through us; we can choose how to play our role; any person can change their stars. How can we evolve cultural attitudes into a healthy alignment? Reproduction is in part an attempt to evolve and adapt to a changing environment, making new ones that are more beautiful and healthy needs to be the intention.

On a physical level, in order to reproduce the human species naturally, we need to have a healthy male and a healthy female. Within each cell of our body are two entwined strands of DNA, one from our mother and one from our father. Those two entwined strands are in a deep embrace, both responding to light energy and glowing away themselves producing energy. There are times when they unwind, separate (go into their caves to do their own personal work as all healthy partners do) and then they recombine, come back together and share the deep embrace.

Problems with fertility and reproductive areas may be an expression of confusion over gender issues and roles we play; this may be at the physical, mental, emotional or spiritual aspects level of expressing our sexuality and gender.

Women are normally fertile for about 4–5 days each month and by the partners getting to know and understand fertility cycles pregnancy can be planned and welcomed rather than playing Russian roulette. In the past, women knew their cycles intimately (measuring body temperature and vaginal mucus consistency facilitates this) and knew how to either avoid or facilitate conception; this was augmented with

eating/applying herbs that either encouraged or prevented implanta-
tion of a fertilised embryo (it has been shown that in indigenous cultures and in primates the females knew the diet and so forth that would
either stop a baby being made or help this to happen rather than using
herbs as abortifacients which is a risky business since in many cases the
level of dose that will make a foetus miscarriage is pretty toxic).

Pregnancy

The mother provides a safe container (the womb) for the baby to grow
in, providing good nourishment and nurture, lots of oxytocin, rest, and
love. The mother also goes through an emotional cascade (which can be
challenging for fathers with no strong community to hold them through
this; it is easier for fathers who have had good mentoring as regards this
aspect of the facts of life). The cascade of emotions is natural; it is how
the baby learns about different emotions but obviously, the healthier
the community in which the mother is being held, the more pleasant
emotional cascades the baby experiences. The mother needs protection
and support from the masculine around her; partner, brothers, uncles,
father, grandfathers, friends. She needs nourishment and nurture from
the feminine around her, a healthy community of sisters, mothers,
aunts, grandmothers, friends. The father provides support, and protection, encouragement. The father needs the same and, guess what, that
is what the baby needs too as it does its own job of remembering its
template and growing well. What happens within embryonic development is the most mind-blowing story ever and a study all of its own. For
example, the gut-brain and head-brain develop from the neural crest,
migrating to where they are supposed to be, but remembering where
they came from and keeping the connection. The heart and thyroid
develop from the same embryonic tissue, and then the thyroid migrates
up into the throat; a beautiful poetic description of how the throat sings
our heart song and when our heart song is true we grow and repair well
(that is what the thyroid is all about).

Pregnancy is a healthy state, rather than a pathology and our present
conventional view of pregnancy, what it requires and the glorious state
that it is has become somewhat tarnished. Another thing that the foetus
does is send stem cells to any damaged tissues in its mother's body; it is
in the interest of the baby to have a healthy mother to provide for it once
it is born. That is one of the most amazing miracles I know of.

Birth

Birth is a stressful event for all involved; whether the birth stress is good or bad depends on several things: how the birth is proceeding (any complications?), the preparedness of the parents, the preparedness of any others present in the birth room and the type of input they give (positive or negative or neutral), the actual birth room setting, feeling supported.

Under extreme stress, our pineal gland produces a substance called metatonin which is also produced in near death and mystical experiences. There is also an elevated production of endorphins; birth can be a magical process and a mystical experience. The baby also produces high levels of metatonin. We can look at our culture's rituals about birth, welcoming in the child, attitudes to the mother and father as they go through the process and compare them with others. In some cultures, no men would be present at a birth, the child would not be taken outside the home for 40 days after being born, and only the most intimate members of the family and community circle would be allowed in to visit the mother and baby. In some cultures, the monumental transition that occurs around the family adjusting to a new arrival is taken seriously. In some cultures, the welcoming of a newly incarnated soul into the community is given due gravitas. In some cultures, the parents and sometimes the whole village start working with the child's energy even before conception; the whole village helps with the pregnancy, with naming the child and much more.

An important part of the delivery is the full expulsion of the placenta. The placental tissue is actually part of the embryo's tissue, and this needs to leave the body of the mother totally too in order for her to regain her integral new identity. Most placental mammals eat the placenta (even the herbivores) and humans used to do it too. It is a gift from the child to help her replenish the resources she has given to the baby as it grows in the womb.

The cycles of maturation

All organisms, and probably all ecosystems go through a natural growth cycle of maturation; we all continue to mature up to the point of death.

Our life cycle starts with conception and the development of the embryo within the womb (or egg, or ovum within the receptacle of the plant, or other equivalents).

We are then born and move through infancy and childhood. As we reach puberty, we move through adolescence. We then become adults. The next developmental stage is that of the parent; even if we do not become birth parents, this is a part of the maturing cycle that all can share in. From parenthood, we move into becoming an elder.

In order to move forward to the next stage of maturity, we need a full and healthy experience of each stage of development in the correct sequence.

Problems arise if our external environment causes us to step into a part of the cycle, we are not yet ready for; the child who is forced into the role of adult or parent prematurely when they perceive that this is a necessary survival mechanism. If we get stuck at a particular stage of development, this will also cause problems. If a parent, or society as a whole, tries to keep us in the child or adolescent stage then we will have a warped maturing. Since adolescence was invented or identified during the Victorian era, our society as a whole would appear to have problems moving beyond this point. Parents may try to prevent their children maturing beyond childhood due to the fact that they have an unconscious fear that the adult is seen to be a threat within our society and therefore if the child matures, they will either be ostracised or annihilated; immaturity can be a survival mechanism too. However, immaturity can lead to a lot of angst and a tendency to close down into survival mode rather than living one's life fully.

We have explored the fact that we are communities, nested personalities, nested ecosystems of cells, or spirit. As we grow and mature, our communities go through normal developmental stages. Brian Weller and Jason Bradford describe the developmental stages of a group of community as being analogous to those of a developing being. They correlate the initial childhood with a stage of forming, as we know children are forming on all levels. Adolescence is seen as correlating to the period of storming within a group, and we have all experienced and witnessed that this is indeed how adolescence can be as the inner council vie to individuate within the family and social structures. If this process is successfully achieved then the next stage of adulthood is seen as norming, the next phase is when we reform and eldership is when we can truly perform; that all seems to make perfect sense to me regarding our inner community, our families, our social groupings, our culture and our ecosystems.

Once upon a time, about 5,000 to 10,000 years ago, we began to forget parts of ourselves and believe in duality, isolation, scarcity, separation. Now we are starting to remember, or perhaps we are being reminded. It is time to listen and listen well to what we have to remember. Due to the times we have lived with some of these messages are like writing in the sand (to quote Riane Eisler); when we hear them, they sound wonderful, hopeful, magical and true, but because they go against what we have been told is real for so long the brightness fades quickly. We need to reinforce our new teachings by feeding them from familiar and unfamiliar sources; heal our hearing and sight defects so that we start to see the world as it actually is. We need to climb onto the lap of our Mother the Earth and listen to her wise stories about how we can grow up to be healthy human beings, in community with our fellow species, our true society of all beings, recognising our individuality but seeing our place and our responsibilities within the community, what gifts and talents we have been blessed with to share with them in order to strengthen the whole and make it more sacred, more whole.

I have been meditating a lot about the times that we live in and the fact that many people are asking what our Mother, the Earth, is asking us to do. The response that came back from many sources was this; our mother is asking us to grow up, to step into maturity. So, then I started more meditating, thinking, reading, asking the council of beings and this is what I heard: the human species is collectively going through developmental stages the same way an individual person does.

When the human species was born or emerged as a species, speciated, or however you wish to put it, it was in its infancy. We are now at the stage of leaving adolescence and moving into adulthood, or rather that is where we should be ...

When an infant is born, they do not perceive any separation from mother; they do not have a separate ego; they have no concept of separation. We have all seen small babies gazing in wonderment at their own fingers and toes. We know that small infants are happiest when they are carried close to the heartbeat of their mother or another close carer as this is what they have known in the womb, the constant entrainment of the maternal heartbeat, the constant intimate connection of being within the mother's body. So, when the human species speciated the individuals, and the collective saw no separation, they kept close to their mother's heartbeat and drew nourishment from her breast—physically, emotionally, mentally, spiritually. They saw no boundaries; they happily engaged with their fellow beings of different species. We have all seen how a small baby that is secure in its parents love, that knows it is truly loved knows no fear. For the first 2 years of their life, an infant's brain patterns are similar to those of an adult when dreaming in the delta range of 0.5–4 Hz; this is described as being the same as the dream or the unconscious state in an adult. In this phase, we are perhaps dreaming our world into being, so although this phase is obviously deeply involved in our physical development perhaps it is also the dreamtime. Perhaps this is why so many cultures have stories and legends about the dreamtime; our species experienced this phase collectively.

Our concept of reality, what we are able to see, hear, sense, the meanings we are able to read from the World, are programmed by our culture during these years. From day 49 of gestation to the age of 3 we produce large quantities of metatonin, our endogenous form of DMT, the spirit molecule, which means that we are continually in a state similar to deep meditation or trance, connected to spirit up to that point. It is possible that this would naturally continue past this point.

Our culture teaches us that we are an individual with a separate consciousness and tends to ignore the concept of connected, collective consciousness. We have touched upon this ultimate paradox before; we are both an individual and also part of the Whole. For most people, by the age of 7, we have become used to our own boundaries of body-self-ego identity and developed the ability to guard the ego, keep ourselves separate; this is seen as the normal mode. Many spiritual practices are about neutralising or quietening the ego, and allowing ourselves to connect to the One, the Universe, the Cosmos; some would say that this is part of our natural being, of maturing; knowing ourselves well enough to be able to experience being individual and not at the same time. Metatonin (endogenous DMT) is the molecule secreted by the pineal gland that enables us to do this. This ability is available to everyone, we all have it, but for many people it is not used. We have already discovered that the skin is intimately involved in obtaining information about our external environment. We sense, listen, with our whole bodies.

A baby will become a toddler and then a child. The child starts to discover ego, strength, their own power and to experiment with what they can do with their strength. A child experiments, learns through play, through contact with the world around them; they explore and investigate and learn. And sometimes they make mistakes and trip and fall, or knock themselves, or put something yucky into their mouths. And sometimes they need guidance or explanations or encouragement to use their strength and power wisely. And sometimes they need to climb on their carer's knee to listen to stories or to be hugged and reassured and have their misunderstandings soothed. And a small child perceives themselves as the centre of their world; if something goes wrong, they will think that they caused it. It takes much reassurance and explanation during their development to remove this error of judgement. We have all heard small children exclaim that it is not their fault and it takes a huge amount of guidance for them to feel secure and mature enough to be able to say 'I spilt the milk' when it was them and 'I did not do it' when they did not, to refuse to take the blame for others' actions and be steadfast in this. A small child needs unconditional love, needs nurture and guidance. I believe that is what we have had from our Mother the Earth.

It has been said that it takes a village to raise a child, the care and guidance of many different mature beings; in the film, *The Man Who Cried*, the female protagonist goes to meet her friend in his Romany community; he has a small child sitting on his lap, and she asks whether the child is his he replies that they are all his children and the old people are all his parents; an extremely healthy answer because our children do not belong to us, they are part of the community. As a species, our guides and carers are the species that were already mature, and our Mother the Earth. We have received unconditional love, but the child needs to recognise and seek this care too. From 2–6 years old, a child spends its time between the delta state and the theta state (4–8 Hz), and this is a similar state to a hypnotic trance or deep meditation. Children are in the imaginal realm at this age. It is similar to those times just as we drift into sleep and when we drift back from sleep in the morning as long as we are not rudely jolted awake by an alarm. In this state, we are highly suggestible and programmable, we really are walking in the Other World. Around 6–7 years of age, we start to operate in the Alpha state as well (8–12 Hz); this is calm consciousness, we start to emerge from our trance with our world view pretty much already programmed (the good news is we can re-programme it later if we do not like what our family, school or culture has taught us to believe).

Childhood has stages, and we all have wounds from our childhood and the human species definitely has wounds and mistakes and misunderstandings that we need to heal; from our individual lives and from our collective past and our ancestral lines. This is part of growing up—seeing the need to do this and being willing to do the work. It takes courage and can feel sore sometimes. However, if we look to our teachers, our guides, our community then we know we have the support we need. If we do not recognise the council of beings as having the gifts and sentience to do this, then we feel isolated and alone—a very frightening place for a child. In *Becoming the Way We Are*, Pamela Levin writes more about the specific stages of childhood, and the part our own inner adult and parent take in us maturing successfully.

Around 12 years of age, the Beta range of brain waves starts to kick in (12–35 Hz), and we develop a much greater ability to focus. As puberty starts a new stage is entered into, adolescence. In The *Gifts of Elders*, Gill Burkett says that adolescence was invented by the Victorians and that ever since we developed the concept we have been stuck that place as a species. Perhaps it is the case that our species needed to go through adolescence and learn the lessons that can only be learned by transitioning through that stage of development. The adolescent stage may be seen as the stage of developing emotionally, but it is important that this is not at the expense of embracing our physicality; too often the adolescent in our modern culture starts to reject their physicality and their bodily functions whilst at the same time feeling drawn deeply into the realm of exploring sexually. However, we may need to accept that we may have been stuck in some shadow expressions of this stage and have come to believe that this is the normal, natural state of being a teenager. The adolescent is going through individuation, finding their own identity and their role in the community. When we look at how adolescence is viewed in Western culture, we can see that this stage is not necessarily valued or supported well by society; the rites of passage that are needed and the mentoring that helps us through this stage is very often absent, many of the adults have never experienced the support needed at this stage and do not remember how to reach into their bones, into the ancestral memories, into our own innate human blueprint to recall how to nurture and guide our young people through this stage.

As we emerge from adolescence, we step into a healthy expression of adulthood, hopefully; this is not an endpoint, our maturing continues as long as we draw breath. Dr Clarissa Pinkola Éstes gives a beautiful description of our stages of development up to and past the age of 100 in her book *Women Who Run With the Wolves*; she tells many sacred stories that gives us some profound teachings about the human condition and how to grow up well as a species. Anyhow, in adulthood we learn to step into responsibility and caretaking, taking practical care and nurturing; it is also the time when we may need to overcome some of our mistakes and wounds from earlier parts of our lives. So it is possible that we are now at the point as a species where it is time to step into adulthood—a scary time, the time when we start to explore what's in the bag, as Robert Bly describes it, and the need to choose to step into the next stage, examining the wounds and mistakes without blame, but with a desire for healing. In early adulthood, we are still in the emotional realm, but we transit into the mental realm. At this transit point we need to be sure that we are integrating the physical and the emotional with the mental so that we do not get stuck in the reductionist, rationalist analytical surface thinking mode of pure mentality where the physical is purely analysed, and the emotional is seen as immature and messy, and feminine attributes are put firmly into the undesirable box for both male and female. We need to remember to embrace our inner infant, child, adolescent; all the parts that are there from our evolution. We need to embrace ourselves as physical, emotional, mental and spiritual beings, masculine and feminine within each of us. We need to remember that in order for a child to grow well, they need a community, a village to nurture them; ours is the council of beings, the invisibles, the greens. We need to remember that a healthy adult recognises the continuing need for their mentors and the support of their community in order to express their individuality in a way that feeds the sacred dream of the community; we seem to have forgotten that we have this beautiful support there and forget to ask them to help us. It is natural for a person to make mistakes as they grow and develop—this is how we learn if we choose to learn from our mistakes. Perhaps what we need to do is to journey to ask what we need to let go of and/or embrace into ourselves in order to do our bit of the growing up of the human species. It can be a joyful experience to do this. It is joyful because then we remember that we are not separated from the rest of the Universe; we begin to see that our sense of separation is perhaps the result of a small epistemological mistake at some stage of our species development, and we can begin to trust that it is possible to find our place in our ecosystem, find our niche and heal the internal wounds that lead us to wound our kin. Truly, the healing that is needed can only be done if we each work on our own small part of the human species and on our own personal and ancestral healing. It is when we stop blaming ('it was the creation of the written word, it was the forging of iron, it was the start of agriculture, the reductionists, Descartes, the invention of nuclear weapons') and look to heal and see that we have the potential to solve the present challenges no matter how we got here that we know that we are truly growing up; yes, it is good to see how we got here, but if we wish to continue to be here as a species, if we wish to see humanity getting to the next level of consciousness we need to grow up. Some argue that the attainment of the spiritual stage of development is only truly achievable in the elder stage, I feel that it is a thread that runs through our development and that at all stages we have some degree of spiritual, emotional, mental and spiritual awareness; how well they are recognised and expressed is to some degree dependent on the maturity of our species and our society or community. It would appear that, at least in the Western culture, we are in an emotional-mental stage evidenced by the emotional puerility of our media, arts and culture, and the mentality of purely abstracted science where reductionist, rationalist, surface analytical thought has allowed the madness of such things as releasing GMO organisms from the laboratory, poorly managed nuclear power, the space race and much besides.

The transition to eldership

Menopause is the climax of a natural transition when the hormones produced in the body change to levels of production such that menstruation no longer occurs. In reality, our hormone levels are continually shifting. In adolescence, we reach puberty and become fertile, able to reproduce. From our early 30s, levels start to alter, and fertility reduces. Peri-menopause may last 5 to 10 years (the climacteric), and menstruation normally stops between the ages of 45–55, although it can occur earlier. After menstruation stops, women may still experience mild symptoms of a monthly cycle such as breast tenderness for a number of years. Menopause is a natural part of our life cycle, not an illness. Some women experience various symptoms, but this is by no means a given. Most of the symptoms are signs of depletion, a need to restore levels of Chi. Depending on the symptoms Yin or Yang tonics may give quicker relief, or sometimes a combination of both or just general tonics. It is a time to review and reassess, look at diet, lifestyle and what might need a bit of support. It is good to ask whether the symptoms speak of depletion in general, or lack of support and protection and what will help address this both in the internal environment and the external one. Hot flushes can be seen as a lack of oestrogen or as a raised sensitivity to adrenaline at moments of elevated emotion and therefore one can look at whether to support the Yin energy with herbs such as *Paeonia, Alchemilla* or whether to give herbs that support the kidney Chi (adaptogens) or whether one needs to work on strengthening the boundaries to reduce sensitivity such as *Urtica, Echinacea, Eleutherococcus*. Heavy bleeding can be a sign of depletion and can lead to depletion and herbs that can help include *Vitex, Geranium sp., Urtica, Alchemilla, Quercus, Achillea, Calendula, Rosa, Rubus*. Irritability and mood swings may respond well to assessing what is irritating and upsetting and using liver herbs to both break down hormones and clear emotional energy can be helpful; these include *Taraxacum, Rumex, Arctium, Gentiana, Berberis sp., Artemisia sp.* (not if there is heavy bleeding though), *Calendula, Cimicifuga, Menyanthes*. Weepiness and emotional lability may indicate unresolved grief amongst other things bitter nervines and other nervines will help the neuroendocrine system and include *Borago, Verbena officinalis, Leonorus, Stachys, Scutellaria, Valeriana, Citrus aurantium flos*. Osteoporosis and osteopenia may be a concern and calcium-rich foods, and herbs will support in this case such as *Rubus, Urtica, Valeriana*. Existential angst at any stage is a normal experience.

Andropause is the name given to the shift in hormones in men. There may be emotional issues that arise in which case bitters, and appropriate nervines are needed. Often there is a reduction in energy or a change in the pace at which one can do one's work, and adaptogens can help support the energy, especially Yang tonic and the ginsengs. Prostate symptoms are an interesting one. One study showed that men in Japan actually have similar physical changes in their prostate but do not get the symptoms of problems with urination; this may be due to the high levels of phyto-oestrogens and seaweeds in their diet or due to a stronger male identity. The prostate is the part of the male anatomy that provides nourishment (a female function) for the sperm. Issues of conflict between the masculine and feminine are stored there too. Herbs that can help improve prostate symptoms include *Epilobium, Seronoa, Urtica diocia radix et fol, Barosma, Betulina*. High blood pressure and high cholesterol indicate a need to support the heart and circulation with herbs such as *Crataegus, Passiflora, Rosa, Achillea, Tilia, Melissa* and to help the liver and pancreas with herbs such as *Stachys, Cyanara, Carbenia, Curcuma, Carduus* (these are all bitters, and the bitter energy is considered to help open the heart and circulation too).

As a child, the gender has an innocent and less defined form; the adolescent/adult can become dualistic in their view of gender, but healthy people embrace both within; the wise elder finds it more easy to make a holistic incorporation of the two, moving between states if they have done their work.

The key inputs for healthy longevity are:

- Not overeating (a marginally above starvation level intake of food); although that is not necessarily true if the following points are taken on board
- Being content
- Having a sense of our life path and following it (those who have had a NDE seem to get this one really focused!)
- A sense of belonging to a community; right relationship
- Drinking coffee and eating rosemary, according to a couple of interesting studies
- Cutting out refined sugar and processed food; if the ingredients on the label do not sound like real food (e.g., maltodextrin, E numbers and so forth) they are not real food
- Staying hydrated
- Healthy movement, whether that is swimming, walking, dancing, gardening, boot camp training or whatever floats your boat
- Getting sufficient rest; both sleep at night (generally 8–10 hours since our body carries out many functions in our sleeping time, as does our mind and psyche, and preferably getting to bed by 10 pm) and rests during the day
- Exercising your mind; and also allow it to rest
- Hanging out with the plants; time in Nature with the green allies

Death

We have touched on the fact that our culture wants to negate death. Our medical industry takes the view of preserve life at all costs; it is about keeping the person alive, rather than the quality of life because that gives greater profits.

In the Tibetan book of the dying (and other equivalents from other cultures), a map is laid out of the bardos or realms that the soul travels through after it leaves this life. It is thought that it takes the soul 49 days to complete this journey and therefore ritual and prayer is offered to help with the transition. In other cultures, the rituals and prayers may not last as long, but there will be time set aside to ensure that the soul successfully moves to the place after death. It would be considered important that the person dies in the right place, Somé recounts the story of his grandfather walking from the mission hospital to his house in order that he could depart well even though he had been in a coma for some time. There would be rituals around family and significant others saying goodbye and ensuring that they were in no way holding onto the person so that they could leave easily. In India sandalwood is burned to help this transition. In other places, frankincense, cedarwood, cypress and other herbs are used. It is said that the soul weighs 21 g.

Rebirth

Apart from the transition from this life onto the next stage, life itself can be viewed as a series of 'little deaths and rebirths'. We all face times of transition—either outer circumstances such as change of job, new relationships, the ending of relationships, moving location, house and so forth, or times when we become aware of inner change (those that occur at certain stages of life such as puberty, andropause/menopause, or simply when we start the process of rigorous self-examination and seeing what serves and what no longer serves). A useful analogy is to look at a mature tree; you will notice that it will from time to time lose small limbs or branches, and sometimes may lose large ones. Deciduous trees let go of their leaves in the winter. When one looks carefully at the trunk and branches, one will notice scars and holes. The tree lets go of the parts that no longer serve but continues to live vibrantly. On a spiritual, emotional and mental level, we need to do the same; we need to reflect and see which ideas, which philosophies, which thought forms, habits no longer serve us if we are to continue to grow and live vibrantly.

Emotional energy and some concluding remarks

Fear alerts us and releases energy (and we can do this without panic), anger releases energy to change the things we do not like (and we can do this constructively), grief helps us to let go of the things that are no longer present or that no longer serve, the heart's joy moves all into the place of unconditional love and healthy passion, willing to do the hard but fun (even joyful) work of being whom we were born to be (ourselves), and singing the Universe, the forest, Nature, the Earth into being day by day, of dreaming the impossible dreams and dreaming sacred healing into being on the face of this planet, the Earth, our Mother and Father; Nature is not just female; healthy Nature contains and embodies healthy masculine and feminine.

So, we find our feet and learn to walk in them, gently and softly, with kindness and caring upon the surface of the planet, in harmony with our fellow beings, with care and compassion.

We let the energy of our hearts flow into our hands, our feet, our heads, our guts, our entire being to do our work.

We receive the loving energy of our fellow beings, and it helps us to generate more of that energy to feedback, the most renewable source (with both oxytocin and love the more that is produced, the more we produce).

We recognise and receive the gifts of the Earth and the gifts of the Cosmos, and we feed those of the Earth up to the Sky and those from the Sky to the Earth, and all the time that means we do the essential human ecological function of transforming fear into love, healing and pouring more sacred medicine into the ancient whole, unseparated, non-dualistic Being. We make it as simple as it is in all its complexity and as complex as it is in all its simplicity.

Gary Snyder (*The Practice of the Wild*) talks of all the unsung unrecognised bodhisattvas, the ordinary ones who do not sit in rarefied settings chanting, removed from the world; he talks about the ordinary ones who get up every morning clean the house, care for the children and elders and sick, who clean roads, mend cars, build furniture, dig gardens and do it all as a prayer to the universe, as a walking meditation, who listen to the songs of the universe and sing them back in the most humble simple settings and ways, this is the true way of the wild, of the indigenous, of healing the interior wounds and so healing the world and the Earth and the Universe. If we wish to heal, the Earth is doing just fine, it is ourselves we need to heal, and our relationship with the council of beings; we must start with that part of the Earth that we inhabit which is ourselves. Forgiveness and forgiving, opening our hearts to allow compassion and devotion to flow out. Shining in a light to see where there is fear or ugliness, demons and monsters. Being aware, present all the time and staying conscious.

The only person we can heal is ourself; we can hold space and pray for others, we can ask is there anything they need, we can (to some degree) eat the darkness and pain for them as they offer it up, we can hold the litter bag for them to put their stuff into, we can help them dig the hole in which to bury their fear to be composted; we can produce a shower of unconditional love to help to wash it away if they are willing to release it, but it is they who do their healing and we who do ours; step into our own power and help them to reclaim theirs, be vigilant of those who shoot in the pins of enchantment, like the tutor in the story of the Maiden King. We are all humans, perfect at being who we are; and work never ends until we draw our last breath (and possibly it goes on after that, but it is different then), we have to accept that we do it each day every day, and some bits have to be done again and again until we get them right, and then sometimes we have to do them again and again because we are good at them and that is what the Universe needs. One day recently I asked the universe: why do I get this work to do, and they said because you are strong, so I asked whether I could be weak; and they said that was not an option, so I smiled, and cried, laughed and got on with it. If we try not to do the work, we end up losing or abandoning our souls; I have seen people go through a deep ego struggle, I have seen people abandon their soul; it is the saddest thing to witness. This is different to putting parts of ourselves in the bag; they can be reclaimed; it is different to soul loss, those parts can be reclaimed; it is different to soul theft; it is different to giving parts of our soul away or taking on parts of other people. Always keep good care of your soul, it is who you are, and we all need to keep our soul in integrity.

The forest

As far as I can see incarnating as a human being is about having fun (respectfully, responsibly, in integrity, with a heart-centred intention, in coherence, community, clear communication, with commitment and all those other bits, obviously); enjoying the sensations of physicality-taste, touch, smell, sight, hearing; about playing; about emotion (not activation and reacting, but pure emotion). Integrity is not just being together enough to do the work, but being completely together, I am learning that one the hard way and endeavouring to find the fun, easy way to do it; some days it works. It is also about pain and grieving, of learning to let go, deal with loss and transition, learning that change is inevitable (except from the vending machine).

These two experiences are not opposites; they can all be experienced at the same time. There is the exquisite agony of being in love; the agony and the ecstasy; laughter and tears together. When I heard that my father was in the process of dying, I went to the forest with my children; I could feel my father was passing on from this existence and I was walking with a full heart. A red squirrel, the shyest of animals and a sentinel of the oak forest, climbed down a tree next to us and grabbed a slice of pan bread that someone had left for the ducks, he hopped over to us, we hardly dared to breathe as he hopped close enough to nearly sit on my son's foot and stared up with his beady bright eyes, then bounded off to the trees with his prize, a wonderful moment. Then one of the deer, a stag, came over towards us and stared deeply into my eyes, seemingly right into my soul in the most reassuring way. I guess I should explain that my surname, according to some, means a grove of oak trees and that the squirrel and the deer, as animals sacred to the oaks, hold a very special significance for me. My father died two days later, peacefully after many years of anguish. One year later, on the anniversary of his death, we decided to go to the forest again to mark the day. As we drove over, it started to pour with rain. When we got there, there was a veritable monsoon. And as we drove back, I swear that I actually drove through about seven rainbows, not under but through the arcs as they touched the earth, pure magic. Later we were sitting at the kitchen table sharing memories of my father, and my 7-year-old son was crying and laughing at the same time, and my daughter and I found ourselves joining in and saying 'Isn't it the best?' Later as I lay in my bed, I could hear the oaks calling as the grief flowed, wishing I could understand.

Yes, we feel the pain of the world, but we don't have to carry it, we walk with it and heal our own wounds; we patiently soften that stagnant emotional energy so that it can flow back to the universal pool, to add it to dreaming the change we wish to bring about. Waiting, not rescuing, just asking, 'Is there anything you need?'

Examples of herbs for the reproductive system

Achillea, Alchemilla vulgaris, Anemone pulsatilla, Anethum graveolens, Artemisia species, Asparagus racemosa, Capsella bursa-pastoris, Carduus marianum, Centella asiatica, Cimicifuga racemosa, Dioscorea villosa, Eleuthroccocus senticosus, Foeniculum vulgare, Glycyrrhiza, Humulus, Lamium, Leonorus, Mentha, Mitchella, Nymphaea, Paeonia, Panax, Prunella, Rosa, Rubus, Salvia, Serenoa, Smilax, Tanacetum parthenium, Taraxacum officinalis radix, Trifolium pratense, Turnera, Urtica, Vaccinium, Valeriana, Verbena, Viburnum opulus, Vitex, Withania, Zingiber.

PART IV

PLANT STORIES

This final section of the book contains 25 conversations with plants that we have growing in the gardens here; some of our interactions with them and the things they have told us, and some of our experiences of using them for healing and food.

Daisy

Bellis perennis Asteraceae.

We have a lot of daisies here because this little plant is a most miraculous healer, and because they bring out everyone's inner child. I remember a couple of years ago sending a group of students out to pick the flowers to make a hot infused oil for salve. When I went out to see how they were doing about 20 minutes later, there they were sitting with happy wee smiles and daisy crowns and bracelets and daisies in their ears and one lying half asleep in the daisies; I think I muttered something ironic about them looking like a bunch of hippy herbal students in mock disapproval. They did all look so very happy, and I have to agree with Julian Barker that it is quite strange how people try to eradicate these beauties from their lawn. About 4 years ago, we began a deep new friendship with daisies. We remembered that they are called bruisewort and wondered how they would do as a replacement for arnica which is expensive, comes from a highly pressured ecosystem and does not produce its medicine well under cultivation (some plants are like that). Also, daisies are native and plentiful. So, we made a warm infused oil and a salve with daisy and plantain with some lavender and tea tree essential oils. The results were miraculous, one of the students got dragged through a fence by her donkey and had really bad bruises, the oil worked wonders. Another used the salve on old acne scars, brilliant results; another gave it to her friend, a chef who finds it clears the burns that are an occupational hazard like nothing else she has tried. It has been used for haematomas, for bites and stings, bruises from rugby practice, sunburn (I would never normally use an oil or salve for this but the people who have tried it got brilliant results). There are so many instances in which it has performed its great healing.

And going out to pick a colander of daisy flowers on a sunny day does not seem like work at all, whether chatting to the daisies or doing it with a couple of comrades. We transplant daisies that pop up in places other than where we need them and give those unfortunate people who have none in their gardens plants to take away. Last year we made an aromatic water from them, lovely and zingy and so refreshing on the skin. The flowers contain loads of vitamin C and are delicious in salads.

I have seen all sorts of interesting recipes for cooking with them. Its Latin name is *Bellis perennis*, probably referring to its beautiful Nature. The name Daisy may well be a corruption of Day's eye as the flowers open and close with the sun. Daisy helps us to see clearly, literally, but also seems to clear our inner eyes of traumatic memories and images that cloud our inner seeing, I have worked with it a lot for that, and helps us get rid of the rose-tinted lenses too. The daisy also seems to help clear the solar plexus, allowing trapped emotional and other energies to release down to the earth or up to the sky. Those flowers with the pink tinge at their edges are so pretty. This is a well rooted and grounded wee soul which really helps to heal childhood wounds and refresh the inner child. In homoeopathy, it is used for wounds from childbirth and for pain relief amongst other things and even clears old birth traumas. This is another dear friend that is bringing its medicine back after being rather ignored for decades and one that sings the song of the strength of our common, native allies most emphatically. I have to say the evidence indicates that it is better than arnica for treating bruises and is a safer remedy to use since it is safe to ingest. It is also useful for bronchitis and bronchial catarrh.

Hawthorn

Crataegus laevatiga Rosaceae.

Hawthorn, which is also known as may or whitethorn, can live for a very long time. The tree grows throughout Europe, North America and Asia. Seeds usually take 18 months to germinate, and therefore it is normally propagated from cuttings. The flowers or flowering tops are usually harvested in late spring around May with or without leaves and need to dry quickly but gently. After harvesting in the autumn dry fruit slowly with a little heat, for example in the hot press.

In Ireland, whitethorns are known as fairy trees, one that connects us to the realm of the invisibles, and woe betide anyone who cuts one down. This is indicative of the value placed in their medicine; so strong is the belief here that planned road routes and building plans have been altered to avoid the removal of hawthorn trees.

Ireland is a country of the heart—all that green everywhere. When the forests were cut down, the wolves were extincted, and the land was taken away by enclosure and given to the landlords, the only tree that peasants were allowed to continue to plant was the hawthorn; hawthorn mends broken hearts (it is a cardiac tonic) and connects us to the other realm. All those hawthorns that burst with blossom in the spring and drip with red berries in the autumn mend broken hearts and are doubly generous as they offer that medicine both in their flowers and their berries.

When hawthorn flowers, in May, it looks like it is covered in icing sugar or confetti, sweet symbols of love.

A superstition arose that it was unlucky to bring the blossoms into the house: 'It smells of corpses, it brings death'. It certainly has a musky scent, but more akin to pheromones than rotting flesh, more allied to the rituals of Beltaine, of fertility and celebrating fecundity and sexuality. But the May tree also mends broken hearts, a very risky business; if people's hearts start to mend, they recover the seat of their soul, they find that passionate ability to fight for their lives and for what they believe in, they wake up and start to see and feel the wounds of the world and feel a desire to heal them.

There is a hawthorn tree in the grounds of Blarney Castle who wraps her branches in an intimate embrace around the ash beside her. They grow so closely that at first, one could mistake them for a single tree; their union is an awesome entwining of spirit. They have lichens on their bark, and the ivy reaches gently up the ash's trunk, gently mind you. In spring we visited them, the love they give into the world is powerful, and they were just waking up from the hardest winter in over 20 years. Myself and the children went to greet them, and the hawthorn drew us close, so close that we found ourselves leaning on her trunks (she has several, so much better to share her medicine with more than one person), we closed our eyes; and then we felt it, so strong, so rhythmic—we had to open our eyes to make sure that she was not actually moving because, as sure as if you rest your head on the chest of someone you truly trust and love, we felt her heartbeat, we heard it with our inner ears. 'Did you feel that?' our eyes were wide with wonder, we lent in again and felt the strong rhythm of her pulse as she was waking up. We could feel all the worries of the world washing away (hawthorn is so good for anxiety, at any time, but especially at midlife), we could feel ourselves entraining with her strong beat (hawthorn will bring the heartbeat and the blood pressure into a healthy place, soothe palpitations, slow tachycardia, restore a regular rhythm in arrhythmias, lower hypertension and raise hypotension); sometimes when she does that work on the heart and circulation all the fluid that we hold onto to dilute our fears and protect ourselves from hurt will be released from the tissues (an initial diuretic effect), and the blood will circulate freely up to our head to feed our brain, so we think more clearly, down to our hands and feet resolving circulatory problems.

The young leaves and flower buds are used as both a food eaten in spring salads and as a medicine. The flowers taste cool and astringent. For medicinal use an infusion or tincture is prepared which has been shown to be valuable in improving the heartbeat rate and strength; it slows heart rate if too high (chronotrophic) and lowers force of heart contractions if too strong and vice versa (ionotrophic). It is especially helpful in heart failure or when the heart is tired from too much strain, whether emotional, mental, spiritual or physical.

Hawthorn helps with irregular heartbeats and improves the peripheral circulation, helping with conditions such as Raynaud's and Buerger's and with poor memory since it improves the circulation to the brain. The bioflavonoids relax and dilate the arteries and blood vessels (it is a vasodilator), thereby relieving angina heart failure and helping the recovery from coronary heart attack. It is also a peripheral vasodilator which can help balance the blood pressure and increase the blood supply to the tissues; the addition of horseradish and or cayenne can be very helpful. Since it improves blood supply to the tissues it has traditionally been included in formulae for treating skin conditions such as eczema and psoriasis and can significantly speed healing time for such conditions; its anxiolytic effect may also be of some benefit here. The bioflavonoids and proanthocyanins are also valuable antioxidants which help repair and prevent tissue damage, especially in the blood vessels; there is evidence to suggest that it can treat arteriosclerosis and can dissolve deposits in sclerotic and thickened arteries. Those antioxidants have also been shown to help with collagen repair.

Hawthorn helps to relieve anxiety and is traditionally thought to mend broken hearts, both emotionally and physically; it is especially helpful at reducing anxiety during menopause and andropause which is a time when many people look back at their regrets and may be struggling to remember who they are, their heart truth.

The berries are gathered in the autumn and have similar medicinal properties. They taste sweet, sour and warm. The fruits can be used fresh or dried in a decoction or infused in brandy (or other spirits) to make a heart tonic for the winter months; both the berries and the medicine made from them have a deep red hue, reminiscent of the colour of healthy blood.

Berries tinctured in brandy have a particular reputation as a winter heart tonic.

For culinary use, the berries are traditionally gathered after the first frost which converts some of the starches to sugars (enhancing their sweet/sour taste) and makes the berries more palatable. Berries are used as an ingredient in hedgerow wine, or to make haw jelly as an accompaniment to wild game. The berries can also be mashed, removing the skin and seeds, and used to make a fruit leather as a way of storing them. Hawthorn was traditionally used to treat kidney and bladder stones until an Irish doctor noticed its benefits for the heart. Even when it is being used as a heart medicine it will often increase urinary output for the first few days as the heart output improves and fluid retained due to poor cardiac function is set the way of the kidneys; it is therefore important to ensure adequate fluid intake (about 1.5 litres a day) and the proximity of toilet facilities.

Elecampane

Inula helenium Asteraceae.

This is an ally I have come to value more and more over the last few years. When I was studying to be a herbalist, this was described as a herb for respiratory conditions, but really this beauty does so much more than that. It is invaluable in the treatment of phlegmy conditions of the lungs, bronchitis, chest infections, asthma, sinus infections and clods but it also works energetically on the lungs to clear old grief and sorrow. Chewing the root is an excellent way to clear the sinuses; the taste is quite intense, a combination of aromatic and bitter, but it really works well.

It is one of our local adaptogens or nutritive tonics (many roots are), supporting the adrenals, spleen and urinary systems as well as the lungs and digestion. It was formerly used as a root vegetable, and the roots were candied as a cough remedy.

As well as treating the lungs it is a wonderful digestive tonic full of inulin which is a good prebiotic. It can help to clear excess mucus in the stomach that can be associated with nausea, distension, flatulence and vomiting.

Inula has been shown to be effective against MRSA and is an effective anti-infectious plant.

It has a history of being used for sciatica and lower back problems, and I can attest to its value in treating these, especially when they come with menstrual issues, for which it can also be helpful.

As a warming bitter, it is very valuable for treating the digestion, stimulating good liver function and warming chilled digestion to help it function better.

The inulin it contains may well help with good calcium absorption and facilitate improved bone strength and health.

The plant may not be native but happily naturalises here and can be propagated by seed or by dividing the roots. It is a joy to grow as it is a perennial with beautiful yellow flowers that look like mini sunflowers. The plants are wonderfully statuesque and elegant.

This plant has become one of my best allies over the last few years and one that I find invaluable in practice. We also make a vinegar infusion of it which has rather a delightful flavour. We recently made an oxymel using this vinegar and honey that had been infused with whole lemons and ginger slices which proved quite astoundingly effective for tracheitis and irritating coughs and sinus infections.

We have also included it in our bitters metheglin, along with burdock, dandelion root, a little gentian and rosemary, plus some cardamom to sweeten it. We have found this improves with ageing for a year or so but certainly is effective as a bitter remedy.

Motherwort

Leonorus cardiaca Lamiaceae.

Our motherwort plants in the garden seem particularly vigorous, and this gives me great hope for the future and the restoration of healthy relationship with Mother Earth and with the mothers in our community who have been so undervalued. The attitude towards the sacred role of the mother in our culture (one of disrespect and dishonour) is reflected in our culture's treatment of the planet. It is disputed whether motherwort is actually a native in this part of the world or a garden escape from the times when it was widely grown in gardens for its medicine. It is however a native of Europe, as well as Asia and North America. It is a hardy soul that will thrive happily in our climate and quickly spread if allowed to seed (mothers are hardy souls, especially when given freedom to express their creativity in most environments). This plant has become a highly valued ally for me both personally and in practice over the last few years. A wonderful medicine is prepared from the aerial parts during flowering. It can be used as a tea, prepared as a tincture, aromatic water, as a syrup and used to make a flower essence. A few years ago, I gave some plants to my friend Carole, who returned a gift of a lovely flower essence she had prepared from them when they flowered with the following suggestions for its use:

('The lion-hearted Mother. Support for Mothers and children of all ages. Assists mothers during traumatic situations with their children as well as healing the mother-child relationship, including the transformation of painful wounds from childhood. Brings courage, integrity and self-belief; reduces tension and anxiety; eases physical pain; restores the heart').

Lions tail or motherwort is aptly named as it is a most valuable ally plant for mothers and children. The plant is sometimes described as a uterine stimulant, and it does help in the birth process. I feel it is more of a tonic and balancer and that it works as a tonic for the sacral plexus as well as the uterus since it is nervine par excellence. Having read about the significance and functioning of the sacral plexus for women's health in Naomi Wolfe's book *Vagina*, I am convinced that this is one area that this mighty ally helps to repair and relax. The alkaloids are the constituents that are key in facilitating labour, supporting women in childbirth since they help facilitate uterine contractions, especially stachydrine which encourages co-ordinated contractions and removes spasms. Some authors say it is contra-indicated during pregnancy, but I know others who swear by its value during pregnancy as support for the woman and baby; maybe this depends on the practitioner's particular relationship with this plant and with the experience of pregnancy and childbirth?

It is also valuable for recovery after childbirth. It can help to encourage menstruation, especially if it is absent due to nervous tension. It also eases period pains that are worsened by tension. Motherwort is also used to treat vaginal infections and discharges. Some authors say not to use with heavy periods unless combined with herbs to ameliorate this possible side effect. I have used it with other herbs such as *Geranium maculatum* or *Robertianum*, *Mentha species*, and *Viburnum opulus* to good effect without any adverse increase of bleeding for women who obviously needed its nervous support during menopause or after childbirth or with heavy bleeding as part of the symptom picture after traumas to the womb.

Its botanical name refers to its ability to give us the courage of a lion, supporting the heart and the nervous system. It is often cited as helping to treat high blood pressure, but it seems rather to balance the blood pressure. It is a bitter nervine that helps us gain calmness and courage in our lives, particularly valuable for the passage through menopause which is a time for self-reflection and evaluation, of clearing and rebuilding as we go through the transformation of our energy into that of the crone which is a kind of rebirthing of ourselves and transformation of our internal and external relationship with mothering as we move forward from the time of our life where we can physically bear children into a different role in our community.

Motherwort is a heart tonic par excellence, some say it lowers blood pressure, but I find it is more of a balancer of blood pressure. It also helps treat tachycardia and palpitations and is good for effort syndrome (where the heart struggles with heavy workloads) and on an energetic level for hearts that feel tired from too much effort and load.

As a nervine, it promotes relaxation rather than drowsiness with this calming effect being due to the bitter glycosides.

Its bitterness makes it a valuable aid for nervous indigestion with wind and bloating. The bitterness means it probably works on the liver, the gut-brain, the heart energy (bitters are used to balance the fire element in TCM) and the vagal tone. It also has some pungency which means that it has the cooling, drying and dispersing the energy of the bitter but also a balancing warmth. I have to say I love bitters and *Leonorus* has a rather lovely taste.

Before sitting down to write about this wonderful healer, I decided to read about her in Mrs Grieve's glorious tome *A Modern Herbal* and found out some new things about this plant that made me toddle off to the dispensary to take a dose. Apparently, it is also good for spinal problems (my back has been complaining about too much lifting in the garden), and it is also good for wet coughs and drying up cold phlegm (I have a residual cough after a nasty cold a couple of weeks ago, and the soggy weather is making it harder to shift all that cold damp from the system).

Grieve also says that Culpeper attributed this herb to Venus and Leo and felt that it was one of the best to drive melancholy from the heart and warm and digest cold humours from the veins, joints and sinews and that Macer considered it all-powerful against wicked spirits.

At this time women are calling to be recognised as equals with sovereignty over their own bodies. Women are calling for the recognition of the value of the unpaid work (my husband says that the overcoming of patriarchy starts in the kitchen and with the housework being equally shared, and that male privilege has to be given up there before we will see equality in other places—we are working on it). The unpaid work of raising the next generation, of taking care of the home, of often caring for the elders. Women are calling for the right to be respected, not treated as objects and servants by those around them. In our culture, we are accustomed to mothers and the earth being seen as resources to be plundered. Women are still not seen as equal; they are objectified in the rape culture; the work that they do is seen as of less value and as mundane—one could say an awful lot about our culture's view of women, the feminine, of mothers and the value of what women have traditionally done in the community. At the same time, we treat our planet, the Earth, atrociously, plundering resources, taking without asking, without giving back, without ensuring that we are respecting, ensuring sustainability, sufficient for the future generations. We worship the machine and curse the genius and miracles of vitality, of life, of Nature. What we can be certain of is that we need to change and change fast so that the children have any hope of a future at all ...

Motherwort is a beautiful, strong ally for the times we live in. May her medicine help heal our relationship with the Earth and with the mothers who bear our children and those that raise our children with unconditional love.

Pine

Pinus sylvestris Pinaceae.

Conifers were rather neglected as valuable allies for a while, but we are remembering them. Pine beer is an old traditional brew that clears the chest and the mind, deepens breathing and settles the digestion. The young buds are juiced in some cultures as they are full of vitamin C and other wonderful spring tonifiers. An infused vinegar of pine or spruce needles or buds is a wonderful alternative to balsamic vinegar, and we use our homemade pine metheglin in winter game stews along with some wild mushrooms and root vegetables.

Pine is an amazing tonic to the lungs and respiration, helping us to breath more deeply and clearly. Pine also has a strong affinity to the HPA (Hypothalamus-Pituitary-Adrenal axis, or endocrine axis). It supports the adrenals and pine oil can be rubbed over the adrenal area to help recovery from stress or withdrawal from steroid medication. Pine also works on the pancreas and digestive area and the solar plexus. I have seen it help to improve thyroid function too as it works on the neuroendocrine system.

It opens the lungs and has a very clearing effect on the pineal gland (so called because it is a similar shape to a pine cone). The pineal gland both produces and is sensitive to metatonin, as well as producing melatonin and serotonin. Metatonin is the mystic molecule, adding meditation and journeying, melatonin gives us calm sleep and serotonin helps us feel good in wake time. Pine also supports the gonads, and pine pollen is a natural testosterone source. Pine helps to strengthen our core axis reaching right from the base roots up to the crown; connecting us from our base right up to our loftiest thoughts and aspirations.

Pine supports our immune systems and is gently warming. Walking in a pine forest (or a spruce one bathes us in negative ions the same way that a visit to the ocean does).

Traditionally, people recovering from consumption (or TB) we sent to convalesce in sanatoria in the pine forests. It is possible that pine could be a valuable ally in both the treatment and prevention of TB which is on the rise. We regularly gather the pine resin exuded from the trees on our local woodland (being careful not to damage the tree and remembering to offer thanks for their generosity). It is one of the things we regularly burn as a fumigant to clear the space from pathogens and also to purify the energies here. We have found this to be extremely effective.

Pine is an ally that deserves a lot more exploration and attention along with other ancient allies amongst our conifer kin.

Rosemary

Rosmarinus officinalis / Salvia rosmarinus Lamiaceae.

Although rosemary is apparently a Yang tonic, I always see her as a feminine ally. She is one of my best friends; I have more than 10 rosemary bushes in the garden each with their own particular personality. About 5 years ago my grandmother rosemary died due to deep freezing conditions in the soil here, and I was sad. One little cutting survived though, and that wee sprig is now a vigorous bush, gaining strength day by day.

Once again, we are enjoying her clear blue flowers in the spring, opening the mind after the hibernation of winter, clearing our thoughts, readying for spring, giving food to any early bees; her deep bitterness that clears stagnant toxic emotions from the liver; her delicious aroma that awakes dulled senses—physical, mental, spiritual.

Rosemary is for remembrance for sure. It improves the circulation to the head and improves memory and is packed with antioxidants which reduce ageing and add tissue repair. It helps regenerate nerves and reduce nerve pain too. It is wonderful for those pale aesthenic young women with low blood pressure and wiry pulses or indeed anyone with low blood pressure and poor circulation. She helps the lifeblood circulate through our vessels when the world seems too cold. It is great for convalescence and for older people. Foot baths with rosemary are wonderful for the circulation. It is also a kidney chi or adrenal tonic, helping strengthen our bases again. It helps when the mood is low, and the energy has all seeped out of the feet, it brings it up again. It is a cordial or heart tonic too. So, it helps the heart, the kidney energy and the brain. It also is good for clearing the liver of stagnation and helping us digest rich food (hence rosemary with lamb, another good yang tonic). It makes the best red wine gravy.

Rosemary is for fidelity; in Italy, they make a wedding bread with rosemary for fidelity and garlic for longevity fidelity and commitment is greatly enhanced by that honest, open communication that comes from the heart and rosemary certainly helps us to do this. It also helps us be faithful to ourselves, the most important factor in healthy relationships as far as I can understand. And looking through some notes from my rather dry herb college days I was astounded to see that one of our lecturers had told us that rosemary binds our souls into our bodies, she does most effectively so can be most valuable when going into trying scenarios or to help the soul return when there has been shock and trauma.

Rosemary can also be burned as a smudge to clear a space and purify the air. Indeed, rosemary and thyme used to be burned in hospitals to keep the air sweet. Rosemary has long been planted in graveyards in memory of the ancestors, she has long been used in smudge and incense to clear space, to create a sacred healing space where open hearts can bring healing to the debilitated worn out body and soul; she helps the soul to be strongly connected into the body, into the heart, its seat in the body.

Rosemary is a cicatriscant and helps repair the skin when it is damaged by burns, wounds or skin conditions like eczema and psoriasis; it also helps dissolve and repair keloid scars and old lumpy scar tissue. Energetically, it will help us to regenerate our boundaries and auric field when it feels rather bashed and scarred.

Rosemary is also a mucolytic, excellent for breaking down thick, sticky phlegm and damp residues in the tissues.

One of the most precious things she has taught me is this; she has been one of my dearest allies for at least 25 years, but I never get to know her completely, there is always more to learn about her multi-faceted deep personality and her amazing powers as a healer.

Elder

Sambucus nigra Caprifoliaceae.

The elder tree (*Sambucus nigra*) is aptly named, a veritable elder and true healer. My friend Siobhan took me to see one in a field near her house. There was a hollow in the field, and an elder was growing in it surrounded by young trees of many species on the slopes around looking for the world like the elder was teaching the young trees how to tree. The elder has much folklore attached to it indicating how valued it has always been for medicine and healing; in several countries, it is reputed to inhabited by the elder spirit, a crone spirit whom one must ask permission of before harvesting any part of the tree otherwise goodness knows what will befall you. It is reputed that if one goes to sleep under an elder tree that one will be whisked off to fairy land and that one should never make a crib from an elder or the baby placed in it will be exchanged for a changeling.

Elder makes many medicines. We use the flowers, the berries and occasionally use the leaves.

We use the leaves to make green ointment which is a traditional salve for arthritis and chilblains and gout. The leaves can also be used as an insect repellent by hanging bunches at the window or over horse stall doors.

The flowers of the elder are excellent at drying up excess mucus, toning the mucous membranes and cooling fever by sweating it out and they open at just the right time to treat hay fever. As well as using them for hay fever we include them in a tea for treating a fever with colds and flus (equal parts of elderflower, yarrow flower and peppermint).

Most of the aroma is in the pollen, and the flowers should be dried out of sunlight and slowly to retain the wonderful aroma and colour. Elderflower is also good for arthritis due to its diaphoretic action which helps sweat out toxins and promote healthy excretion via the skin.

The tea has a reputation for treating candida, and I often recommend it for those endeavouring to balance their gut flora. It is a lovely one to give children and babies with oral thrush and can also be used to bathe the skin to help with dermal thrush.

According to Glennie Kindred, the tea of the flowers is particularly good for those who get anxious in the evening, and it has a reputation for calming fretful babies and children too. One pleasant blend for evening use is elderflower, red clover, and linden blossom.

A hydrosol of the flowers is known as *Eau de Sureau* in France and used as a skin tonic, particularly after shaving. The berries come in the autumn in time to give a good boost to the immune system. They have been shown to be more effective than *Echinacea* for treating colds and flus, and I always leave some for the birds to help their immune systems through the winter. They make an excellent syrup for a winter tonic. The high levels of proanthocyanidins also make elderberry good for collagen and nerve tissue repair and mean that they help to strengthen the blood vessel walls. The berries can have a laxative effect but are also used to treat diarrhoea.

The leaves and bark are no longer used internally by most herbalists, although the bark used to be used as a strong liver tonic.

Tilia

Tilia x europea Malvaceae/Tiliaceae.

It was summer; my heart was hurting from the place of a small child who had reached out into the pain of the world and felt it burn too hot; she was feeling angry, scared and hurt all bundled into one complex emotion ball. My nose was running with all the uncried tears of feeling rejected, of experiencing the anger of others that arises from their fear especially their fear of bliss, so that they lash out. I had been walking with the trees, feeling their medicine and the tears had flowed a little, easing my pain. I followed my children in their carefree playing hide and seek, their feral uninhibited dance with the greens and the invisibles—'Look, here's eyebright!' one of them said, 'it's thyme-leaved speedwell' I found my inner academic replying—I felt like a 4-year-old who was in that awful isolation of grief, so alone. I wanted Mother to soothe me. And then it hit me, like breathing in liquid sunshine, honey-nectar; an aromatic cloud of the scent of the lime blossom, overwhelmingly soft, nourishing, cooling, calming all that irritation in my heart. The anger of others washed away (*Tilia* lowers cholesterol and clears the blood vessels of atheroma), the overheat of my heart cooled and calmed (*Tilia* calms hot flushes and lowers blood pressure, especially when there is nervous tension as well), my nose cleared (*Tilia* soothes the mucous membranes and skin, reduces catarrh, calms irritated guts). My head felt calmer (linden is good for any kind of headache and tension in the head, including migraines. It also calms the mind and allows us to relax). My body relaxed, the tension ebbing away (she's so good for nervous irritability, you know that frantic energy of the child of any age who has gone past the place of being able to relax and sleep, when sleep will not come because of over-stimulation), my shoulders lifted as my heart space opened—I found myself smiling gently, sighing as my heart relaxed, starting to hum, my steps lightening, moving into the rhythm of the children in their wild and free games. And my ears heard the drone of hundreds of bees feeding on the blossom of the lime tree, calm, doing the work at their own pace, no hurry. Linden also releases hysteria and panic and is invaluable for treating panic attacks and nervous palpitations. *Tila* is one of those amazing allies that is cooling and warming, depending on what the tissues need.

It cools the skin and is used in France to make a lotion or wash for irritated and itchy skin in combination with marshmallow. It is also used for bites, boils, burns and sore eyes. It helps to clear feverish colds and flus, and a cold infusion of the flowers can help relieve hot flushes.

At the same time, it can be used as a remedy that is warming and relaxing to the digestive tract; releasing tension and soothing the gut lining due to the mucilage it contains.

Since it contains both mucilage and tannins, it can soothe or astringe, depending on what the tissues need.

It contains antioxidants such as quercetin, kaempferol, caffeic and other acids. The essential oil (mainly farnesol) and benzodiazepine-like substances act on the nervous system to calm and soothe. In addition, it contains saponins and sugars.

Linden blossoms are collected in the summer as they open and release their enchanting aroma. They smell truly beautiful and are much loved by bees for gathering nectar. Their taste is wonderfully aromatic (reminiscent of honey) and mucilaginous.

Valerian, all heal

Valeriana officinalis Caprifoliaceae.

For me, valerian has been a literal lifesaver on several occasions. Although some people are a little wary of this ally myself and the community here, have found that it is a most dependable and trustworthy ally (unless you have a very hot constitution), but the skill is in finding the optimum dose for the individual person.

Usually, the roots and rhizomes of plants at least 2 years old are harvested in the autumn. One of my colleagues suggests growing it in large pots to facilitate harvest, which is a great idea. When harvesting it is possible to divide the plants or take root cuttings so that the harvest of the roots is not entirely destructive. Valerian also self-seeds quite freely, so it is easy to ensure that harvesting does not decimate the population. Henriette Kress says that the aerial parts can also be used, but they are not as strong in their action. We did make an aromatic water from the flowering tops when some lodged over in a storm earlier this year, but we found it to be much weaker in action. However, the flowers have a lovely indole heavy scent reminiscent of jasmine, and that is medicine in itself on a walk in the garden or other places where this plant grows. The bees certainly seemed to enjoy feeding on them too.

Valerian is native to Europe and Northern Asia and cultivated in Britain, Holland and Belgium. It will grow in damp shady woods, hedges, ditches, wet grassland, fens, dry grassland, scrub, woodlands and meadows and it is not difficult to spot it around the countryside. However, in deference to those wild populations and the other species that use it, it is better to sow seeds or buy plants of this wonderful ally to establish a colony in your own garden, if you have one.

Valerian tastes bitter and camphorous, or deliciously earthy depending on your point of view. The smell (due to isovalerianic acid) is supposedly reminiscent of tomcats; cats are attracted to it by another component, an iridoid called actinidine and get quite stoned on it. Apparently, it also attracts rats, and the Pied Piper is reputed to use it alongside his alluring pipe playing to lead the rats away from Hamlin.

Valerian is widely used in relaxing tea blends and to prepare apple flavourings for the food industry. It was known as all heal in the past, showing how valuable a plant ally it was felt to be. It is an incredible healing ally, even having a reputation for curing epilepsy. The name may be from valere the Latin to be healthy or valuable or named after a Roman physician Valerius. It is variously described as a sedative or a stimulating nervine. It is wonderfully anxiolytic and brings the energy down from the head, helping to ground and earth anxiety, panic and whirling thoughts. It is rich in calcium and nourishes and calms the heart too. It would appear to help calm the entire nervous system and all the brains as well as relieving tension in all body systems.

Formerly its sedative action was thought to be due to the isovalepotriates and then due to valerianic acid; now it is thought that it is due to a complex of several constituents.

Valerian prolongs action of inhibitory neurotransmitters, blocking our response to excitatory neurotransmitters and therefore reduces excessive nervous activity. This means that small doses can actually improve focus, concentration and physical performance. It is also splendid in small doses for preventing stage fright, exam stress (I regularly give it to people to take before their driving test and their final clinical exams) or for social anxiety or panic attacks. In these cases, I give it in a dropper bottle so that people can take it as frequently as they need and vary the dose depending on the situation. Often people find that having something to help the anxiety is enough to stop them from experiencing it. It can also relieve nervous palpations and sweating and is excellent for anxiety in menopause or andropause. I find it helpful for people who are experiencing anxiety as a result of drug withdrawal or excessive alcohol intake too.

Valerian is recommended for hypochondria, or for those who constantly worry about their health or feel rather unwell due to constant worry. It is a mild anodyne or painkiller, well actually it can be quite a strong one. I have used it for tooth pain, pain after tooth extraction and for various kinds of back pain, including trapped nerves and spasmodic pain. It also helps relieve neuralgia.

Some describe it as a hypnotic, aiding sleep. Valerian can improve sleep quality and duration and encourage sleep to occur easily but is better taken as several small doses throughout the day, relaxing tension and anxiety rather than one dose before bed. However, valerian is a heating herb so can cause a hungover feeling in those who use it for sleep and who are chronically dehydrated. As a heating herb, it does not suit people with a lot of heat in their systems and can actually cause agitation rather than relaxation in such people.

Valerian is a spasmolytic, relaxing tension in both skeletal and visceral muscles. This may well have added to its reputation as a panacea since it can help bronchospasm in asthma, bronchitis and irritating coughs. It can relieve high blood pressure by relaxing the blood vessels. It can relieve spasm and pain in the digestive tract (intestinal colic, IBS, spastic colon, nervous indigestion) where its bitter and carminative properties also help. It helps with cramps and muscle spasms in the skeletal muscle, relaxing over contracted muscles; this means it can help relieve pain in injured tissues or in arthritis where the muscles are contracting to protect a damaged joint. It will also relieve period pain.

As a digestive bitter and spasmolytic it can help with migraine and tension or nervous headaches.

Valerian is a definite nutritive tonic, rich in calcium which supports the heart, the nervous tissues, the muscles and aids tissue repair.

It has also been used for fevers although I would not think of it as a go-to herb for this, but my husband has found it good during a bout of the flu with the accompanying aches and agues.

Although it is apparently only to be used as a medicine one of my students made amazing scones with a small amount of valerian combined with elderflower and elderberries as the flavourings. It has also been used to manufacture apple flavourings for the food industry.

Marshmallow and the mallow family

We have common mallow (*Malva sylvestris*), marshmallow (*Althea officinalis*) and musk mallow (*Malva moschata*) plants growing here and sometimes a couple of other types. Marshmallow sweets used to be made by candying the roots of that plant, a far cry from today's version. Several years ago, my friend Cathy Skipper came to visit and co-teach a summer workshop on medicine making; she is a very dear soul. We made a flower essence at each day of the workshop, deciding which plants to work with was such fun. Common mallow stood forward; one of the participants at the workshop had lost her mother a couple of months before very suddenly and to see her sitting with the plant with the rest of the group was so touching, one could see the comforting mother energy from the mallow reaching out to her, and she quietly shed tears. When the group fed back about what they felt the plant worked on it was a consensus that it was like mother hugs, warm and reassuring. Common mallow is more short-lived than the other two. We use the leaves of this and of musk mallow in soup, they make a rich, creamy soup due to the large amounts of mucilage; one student asked whether there was cream in it (she was concerned as dairy intolerant), but it gives that richness in a vegan soup, and is so soothing to the digestive tract and nourishing at the same time. That really sums up mallow medicine nourishing and soothing, real mama energy. When my kids were young, they were allergic to sugar and cow's milk (they gave them eczema)—sometimes on a visit to friends they would end up eating some, and if that happened, they would go and gather marshmallow leaves themselves to put in the bath. Marshmallow leaves are rather furry which is why I do not tend to cook with them, although they are OK in soup. The leaves and flowers of the other two mallows are wonderful in salads. Their seed heads are known as 'bread and cheese' and are nibbled as a richly nourishing snack. We used to make a complex formula called intestinal corrective powders with about five powders in it to treat constipation and diarrhoea, now I just use marshmallow root powder, sometimes with a little fennel powder mixed in; this can be grown and produced locally and is far cheaper and more abundant (the other ingredients were green clay of which it is impossible to obtain edible grade at present, apple pectin which is very expensive, and slippery elm which is expensive, not local and the trees are suffering from something similar to Dutch elm disease). Marshmallow root powder also makes a wonderful drawing poultice for boils, carbuncles, abscesses and blackheads. It is a nourishing convalescent food, and one can make delicious brownies with it or mix it into porridge or make face pack mousse (this is a vegan mousse that was originally conceived as a face pack but turned out to be a really nice fruit mousse with berries, honey, ground oats and rose water). It soothes and repairs the gut lining and draws out toxins too, great for diverticulosis and many other conditions. The leaves are used to soothe cystitis, bronchitis and other inflammations of internal linings to the organs; they do this by a reflex action through the gut lining as all these linings are from the same embryological origin and soothing the gut causes the others to calm too and also calms the skin. It is only recently that I have realised that marshmallow root and all the mallow leaves can have a profoundly healing and soothing effect on the lining of the womb, I'm really rather slow sometimes, but it was not taught in our repertory as being good for that too, and unschooling is a really valuable process to go through sometimes, learning the parts one was never taught and unlearning the false lessons. That's just a brief introduction to mallow medicine, needless to say bees love feeding on them too and there are many other stories to tell, but they sure bring a soft gentle but strong energy to the garden.

Apple

Malus species Rosaceae.

When the apple blossom opens, I get very excited, it is so beautiful. Some people pick the blossoms to eat, but I prefer to leave them as valuable food for the bees and cross my fingers for a few dry and still days so the bumbles can do their work and get good food; the sight of them is good enough food for the soul. Apples are the most amazing medicine; anyone who has studied with me laughs when I mention stewed apple and cinnamon as a medicine as it is rather a cure-all as far as I can see. The crab apple or wild apple is one of the Nobles of the Wood in Brehon Law, speaking of its level of esteem and value. Apples are a tonic to the digestion and the liver partly due to their sour taste as sour tastes also tone the liver. Apples are wondrous nutrition full of vitamins, minerals and much more which makes them an ideal food for growing children, those studying or those convalescing, or for anyone really. They contain a substance called pectin, which is even more valuable when cooked. Pectin soothes the digestive tract and draws out toxins and heavy metals; it is so effective that apple pectin has been used for those in the Chernobyl region to help remove radioactive caesium from their bodies but is equally good for drawing out lead or mercury or aluminium. Pectin also helps lower cholesterol and will also bind cholesterol in rich meals (hence apple sauce with pork) so that it is not absorbed. As well as soothing the gut lining and absorbing toxins pectin is germicidal which makes stewed apple and ideal food to give for diarrhoea- even better with some cinnamon and live yoghurt. It is a prebiotic so helps re-establish healthy gut flora. It is also valuable for constipation due to the soluble fibre it contains. Apples are great food for debility or recovery from overexertion. Sour apples are also effective for urinary tract infections. The fruit contains flavonoids, especially if the skins are eaten too, these help with cholesterol and with prevention of stroke and can lower high blood pressure. Apples are also used for respiratory conditions, rheumatism, gout, morning sickness and much more. Apple cider vinegar and verjuice are wonderful fermented foods which deserve a post of their own. Apple poultices can help with poorly healing wounds. Stewed apple at the start of a meal can soothe diverticulosis, colitis and amelio, and rate the effects of food intolerance (unless one is intolerant of apple).

Apple leaf and bark can be used as astringent medicines. We made an aromatic water of leaves and bark combined after pruning the trees this summer. Their aroma of taste is just like stewed apple; it is beautifully refreshing and soothing to the digestion. The Greeks viewed the scent of apple as a panacea, and we really felt that the aroma of this water made us feel healthier.

The apple tree is central to many Paradise myths—the Garden of Eden to name but one. The apple trees is a tree of knowledge and wisdom but also of love, for others and also for self. It helps to harmonise the masculine and feminine and to bring about the development of trust. The apple tree is central to Celtic culture—the silver bough was cut from an apple tree and had nine apples upon its branch that played continuous music and lulled people into a trance or allowed them to journey to the Otherworld. If you only have a small space get a dwarf apple tree and grow it in a large tub; if you have enough space plant an apple orchard, the trees really do exude their harmonious energy and love. In some parts of the world, apple trees are thanked for their gifts of fruit by wassailing—a beverage is prepared for the trees and given to them in the winter to ensure a good crop the next year. I could write a lot more about apples and apple trees ... they are beautiful beings.

Plantain

Plantago lanceolata et major Plantaginaceae.

Harvesting ribwort plantain leaves for our lunchtime salad and seeds to dry to add to our bread is one of those pleasurable summer activities. Plantain leaves have a mildly mushroom flavour probably due to the mucilage they contain. Plantain is also known as waybread since it can be used as a survival food and as white man's feet since it spreads so prolifically. It is related to psyllium, and the seeds have similar uses. It is one of the nine sacred herbs of the Druids and one of the herbs of St. John's eve. It is known as the healing herb in Gaelic due to its wonderful healing abilities for wounds and bruises. We combine it with daisy for a salve to treat wounds and bruises. As well as healing it is antiseptic and can help clean out infection in wounds. It contains allantoin (as does comfrey) which speeds healing but has the advantage of also fighting infection. I have seen it help heal staphylococcal skin ulcers. It is also great for mending damaged tendons and ligaments both in poultices and internally and has the advantage over comfrey that we are still allowed to use it internally. I used it in combination with comfrey externally for a badly sprained ankle a few years ago and could really feel the plantain getting down into the tissues and fixing away. Plantain syrup is still in the official pharmacopoeia in Russian medicine.

Plantain is slightly sweet, bitter, salty and mainly cooling. The combination of mucilage and tannins means that it can be both moistening and drying. When my kids were young, they used to put a few leaves in the freezer ready for rubbing on nettle stings. I find it superior to dock for soothing nettle stings. It is excellent for treating inflammation in the gut, the urinary system and the respiratory system (bronchitis, sinusitis, laryngitis and much more). A tea can be used to bathe sore eyes, and it can also be used for ear problems. The leaves can be placed in the shoes or socks to prevent blisters and keep the feet fresh. In Welsh herbal medicine, it is used as a drawing herb. Plantain modulates the immune system and does much more besides. Energetically, it helps us root down and connect to the earth and to repair our terrain and connection to the land. It is also good for those times when we need to just hunker down and become more mundane. We use the leaves in salads, stir-fries and to make pesto (really nice combined with some sorrel in the pesto); food uses like this are really valuable when people need large doses to help with tissues repair. There is so much more that could be said about this modest humble but incredibly strong healer. It is one of those plants that has really taught us about the miraculous healing abilities of the allies just outside our door in recent years.

Nettle

Urtica dioica Urticaceae.

I love those allies that just spring up outside the door and prove to be the best food and medicine. Nettles are not just great for us; they feed other plants (one can make a wonderful liquid fertiliser from the leaves and add them to the compost to activate it). They are also really important food for the caterpillars of some of our native butterflies. They used to be dried as winter fodder for livestock and have a higher protein content as dried fodder than *Lucerne*.

When the first flush emerges, it's time for nettle soup and raw nettle pesto. My friend Cathy Skipper showed me how to fold and roll nettle leaves so that they can be munched raw (good to have some plantain to hand the first time you try in case it does not go quite right) and they taste quite delicious; she also explained that the juice within the leaf neutralises the sting on the hairs on the leaves so this is why they can be made into pesto, and it is quite delicious and the best blood cleanser and builder. The tradition with nettle soup is to have three feeds of it before May is out to keep one strong and healthy. Once the plants go to flower, they are not so good to eat, and they get stringy and rather high in silica but can still be used for tea. I have patches of cut and come again nettles throughout the summer so that they can be used over the entire season. But I leave some to go to seed as nettle seed is an amazing energy food, tonifying the kidneys and adrenals and full of essential fatty acids, brilliant winter food and as good as those superfood seeds. Some people find picking the seeds a little challenging because of the stings that have to be endured but our friends Fred and Natascha gave us a great idea this summer which was to use a couple of those Scandinavian berry picking combs to comb them off. The roots are full of phytosterols and are a great treatment and preventative medicine for prostate problems. So, what are the aerial parts good for? The Romans used to beat their arthritic joints with them to cause counter irritation and give relief from the condition. Nowadays most people just drink the tea instead. Nettles are anti-histamine, good for hay fever and eczema; they are also high in certain neurotransmitters so are doubly helpful if the eczema is made worse by stress. Nettles help build the blood, they are good for anaemia, being high in iron. They are also high in other minerals such as magnesium and potassium. They can help treat both heavy periods and nosebleeds. They can relieve insect bites when taken as a tea or used as a wash. And they are great for water retention and poor kidney function. They are also amazing medicine for the liver, clearing stagnant there too—all in all a great cleanser. In addition, they contain quite a lot of serotonin which only reaches the gut-brain but can cause an interesting reaction in people who already have high gut serotonin; serotonin does not cross the blood-brain barrier, so this serotonin does not reach the head-brain. They are great for iron during pregnancy too. The finest linen used to be made from nettles, not flax. There is a wonderful old Irish story about the sister who weaves nettle shirts for her brothers who have been enchanted by an evil sorceress and turned into swans. The shirts have to be thrown over them to turn them back into humans, but she runs out of fibres, and so one of the shirts only has one arm, and one brother ends up with one arm and one wing for the rest of his life Nettle medicine is valuable for strengthening and repairing psychic boundaries.

Wild garlic ramsons, bear garlic, buckrams, wild garlic, broad-leaved garlic, wood garlic, bear leek

Allium ursinum Amaryllidaceae.

The sight of the ramsons emerging in the spring gladdens our hearts and gets our mouths watering. The first taste of it seems to spread viriditas tingling into every cell rejuvenating the tissues and the palate after the heaviness of the winter. And when those star-shaped flowers burst open they are a wonder to behold.

Although some people use the bulbs as well as the leaves and flowers, we only do this if some has self-seeded in the path or another inappropriate place. Ramsons is a native perennial plant. It prefers moist and slightly acid soils and occurs in woodlands (it is an ancient woodland indicator plant, along with cow wheat and sanicle), shaded hedge banks and shady stream banks. It is propagated from seed sown in the spring or by dividing clumps and planting them in spring or autumn. If harvesting from the wild, then it is more sustainable to harvest the leaves and leave the bulbs to regenerate for the next season. When harvesting it is important to identify the plant correctly since people have confused it with *Convallaria majalis* (lily of the valley), *Arum maculatum* (cuckoo pint/lords and ladies) or even *Colchicum autumnale* (Autumn Crocus). The definitive factor for correct identification is the garlicky aroma which none of the others possesses; the whole plant has a garlicky aroma; if it does not smell of garlic it is not ramsons; also the time of year of harvesting, it does not emerge in the autumn.

The Latin species names indicate that it is a bear medicine and one of its common names is bear's garlic as brown bears love the bulbs and dig them up; wild boar and badgers also enjoy them. Barker says that the name is due to the bears and the plant having a similar smell and that it is also known as badger's flower in certain areas because of a similar aroma from the plant and that animal. It has a long history of use as a food plant and is used in soups, stews, steamed as a vegetable, added to salads or to make a pesto. It has also been used as a fodder crop for cows and will give the milk a slight garlic taste and smell. There has been little or no clinical research into the use of the plant, but it has a strong tradition of use; according to Brigid Mayes, 'Tagh O'Quinn 1415 mentioned it as hot and dry in 2nd degree use and that only the flowers should be used for medicine. Once prepared it has 2 years shelf life viscous phlegmatic humours cleared'. Barker suggests that its actions are more noticeable on the guts than on the respiratory system.

It contains a volatile oil, vinyl sulphide, aldehydes, and plenty of vitamin C. Its actions are similar to garlic but probably not as strong and definitely not as heating. In the spring it is a valuable tonic, clearing mucus from the system, encouraging sweating, thinning and cleansing the blood, and promoting good digestion whilst clearing acid toxins due to its diuretic effects. It also clears parasites from the gut, including threadworms, candida and amoebae.

As a food-medicine, it has a reputation for protecting the cardiovascular system, balancing blood fats and sugars, balancing the digestion, cleansing the gall bladder, and helping with weight loss.

As a circulatory stimulant, it can help with arthritis, rheumatism and gout. It has also been used in poultices for boils and abscesses.

Wild garlic pesto

Take 1 litre of loosely packed leaves, a cup full of pine nuts, ground almonds or cashew nuts, a small amount of sea salt to taste, 1–2 dessertspoons of vinegar or lemon juice and enough oil (hemp or olive) to make the desired consistency. Place in a pestle and mortar or food processors and pulverise until a smooth paste is achieved. Spoon into jars and cover with a little oil. It will keep for up to two weeks in the fridge.

Burdock

Arctium lappa Asteraceae.

Burdock is one of our native adaptogens or nutritive tonics which cleanses (the liver, bowel and lymphatic system) at the same time as nourishing us (our blood, digestion and immune system in particular).

254 CONVERSATIONS WITH PLANTS

The roots are used as a vegetable in Japan (known as gobo) and used like any other root vegetable—they have a bitter, sweet, nutty, earthy flavour and must be harvested in the first year of growth as they are woody after that. The roots contain inulin and therefore are a good prebiotic for our gut flora. It is a biennial, producing a rosette of leaves in the first year then shooting up to produce leaves the size of elephant ears. The leaves can be eaten as part of a spring cleanse but have a particularly strong bitter taste; I love bitters but find I can only nibble a little piece of these leaves. The flowers are purple, similar to thistle and followed by the classic burrs that catch in everything and are what inspired a French chap to invent Velcro. Those seed heads speak of its ability to comb out old dark thoughts and residues in our physical body too. The seeds can be used for the immune system, and I want to gather them to experiment with them as a native seed food this year, probably full of good essential fatty acids. The seeds have been shown to help prevent cell mutation. To me, this majestic plant helps us to comb out the learned beliefs so that our indigenous, authentic self can re-emerge and fill us up again. There is so much more to this plant's story and personality, but the best way to learn from the plants is to go hang out with them yourselves and listen.

Miracle leaf, love plant

Kalanchoe pinnata Crassulaceae.

Although most of the plant allies we work with are natives of this part of the world we have a few allies that we nurture inside which come from the Caribbean where my mother hailed from. They are rather treasured friends and sing to me of that homeland.

So, this beauty needs to be grown inside in Ireland during the winter as it is originally from the Southern Americas but it is a very close ally for me, and we have shared some amazing times. I first met this plant when I was visiting Trinidad with my mum about 12 years ago on her last trip to the Caribbean. We were visiting my aunt and uncle. My aunt knew about my love for plants and pointed out one of these on her balcony and said it was miracle leaf or love plant (it has many common names, and its botanical name is *Kalanchoe pinnata*). My aunt had used a poultice of it to remove a pre-malignant skin growth. She said that one could take one of its leaves and just leave it in between the pages of a phone directory and that the plant's capacity to regenerate is so miraculous that it would sprout a new plant out through the pages of the book. She gave me a leaf and told me to bring it back home and see if it would grow. I put the leaf in the book I was reading, and the next day we returned to Grenada, and I came home a few days later. The leaf looked rather wilted, so I put it in a cup of water to re-hydrate. Someone mistook this for the leftovers of a herbal tea and washed the cup, leaf and all in hot soapy water. I found it and was sad because I felt that might all have been too challenging, but I took the leaf and laid it on moist compost. Every day I checked it and sent it love. The leaf shrivelled and shrivelled, and I was sad. Then, one day I checked, and truly miraculous a tiny baby plant was forming on the remains. Over the course of time, it grew and grew until it was about 4 foot tall and filled a whole window. At this stage, it became a bit big for its pot and sort of toppled. So, I took lots of leaves and gave one to each of the kids at the primary school next door. Over the course of time, the plant has produced so many babies, and they have been sent out into the world. I always thought of it as a plant to sit with, a plant that would clear a space and one that seemed to evoke a strong oxytocin love response in people when they sat with it; there are so many stories of people sitting with it and describing a journey of coming back to feeling at home in themselves or that pure innocence of the child who feels safe and loved and at home in Nature and much more besides. I read up about how it is a panacea for so many ills to treat the blood the pancreas, the lungs, to heal wounds and so many things. It was only last January that Lucy suggested we try using it to make medicine, I'm a bit slow sometimes. So, she made an amazing skin cream which has been used for some really tricky cases. And, of course, then I drank the leftover infusion and felt it clearing some troublesome winter aches and pains. Since then we have been tending a few mother plants with the intention of exploring its medicine more (and lots of them got given away again) and this spring and summer I look forward to some of them growing big enough again to explore more. I have called it a miracle leaf most of the time but it definitely a plant of green love too, showing the miracle of regeneration after near annihilation and such a generous giving and sharing into the world. Last year, on my birthday, a friend put up a video of a Jamaican herb woman in her beloved rain forest and I squealed with joy (I don't do that often, the squeaking that is) much to the kids hilarity as the video showed her bending into a huge Kalanchoe in her beloved rainforest and speaking lovingly of her relationship with this amazing healer and her working with the plants to bring people into sustainable living and protecting the forest; much like my vision of what is possible here. That's just a brief version of what the miracle leaf has brought into my life, a true friend.

Angelica

Angelica archangelica Apiaceae.

The season of dream mending, I love this phrase; the winter season of the bear in the cave where we mend what we need to through our dreams and mend our broken dreams so that we emerge in the spring re-invigorated, rejuvenated, with new vision and strength for the future. When bears emerge from the cave, they dig up roots to get their digestion and excretion going again (osha, lovage, ramsons). *Angelica archangelica*'s roots are also one of those medicines that help fix our dreams, get our blood circulating again, deepen our breathing, warm our digestion, tone the kidneys and bowel. It is one of the best teacher plants; its very form describing so clearly what it does. The stems have deep red stripes, telling us of its work on our circulation, the big leaves spread out like fully expanded lungs responding to the air, the roots go deep into the soil as an anchor that feeds deeply in the soil, and the flower heads are like haloes denoting how it protects and repairs our psyche, helping us to release trauma (like orange blossom, similar constituents and aroma) and set stronger boundaries. The seeds have a warming aromatic oil; all the parts of the plant gently stimulate our nervous system helping us to concentrate and think more clearly and clearing bugs from the system (literally and metaphorically). It just shouts its message out or sings it like the best ever soul singer. It is sweet and bitter and sour and pungent and salty; all five flavours balancing our energies. Yes, I am totally entranced by this plant. They grow for 2–3 years then seed and die. The seeds are really difficult to germinate if dried but will germinate well if allowed to fall from the mother and grow around her. We got about 300 seedlings from one plant a couple of years ago. The myth goes that humans were taught of its medicine by Archangel Raphael; it was formerly known as the root of the holy ghost. It also treats migraine, anorexia, catarrh, and can be used in compresses for thoracic pain. It is a great restorative for the female reproductive system; although the Chinese species has a bigger reputation for this, the European one is also good medicine in this respect. It is a real medicine chest of a plant and totally beautiful to boot. Our native species *Angelica sylvestris* is more bitter and less aromatic but is still a great medicine. It is a perennial and grows in damp places and is rather more purple in its colouring.

Selfheal

Prunella vulgaris Lamiaceae.

She is one of those most wonderful friends. The last 3 years have been a real journey with her for myself and with the students here. We started by making a tea and noticed how calm we felt. Then people asked whether she could be used in food; a wee exploration uncovered the fact that she is one of those forgotten pot herbs and now she goes into green soup, salads and green omelettes regularly. She is very adaptable, growing happily close to the ground in closely mown lawns but if given the change will spread and stretch up to about 30 cm. She is much loved by bees and used across the globe. In China, they use the flowering heads for cooling the liver and for treating fevers. A wee dram of the aromatic water we prepared last summer certainly helped with the feverishness of a fluey cold. In this part of the world, it has a great reputation for colds, flus and sore throats. After we started to get to know her, we decided to do a co-distillation of *Prunella* and feverfew to make an aromatic water. The art of co-distillation has been a little forgotten, but it helps the energies of the two plants to mingle their healing, and that water was tremendous; the zingy quick clearing energy of feverfew combined with the steady, grounded earthing energy of *Prunella* so that things move out smoothly; we had fun with that one. Last summer we decided to distil *Prunella* by itself, and it is doing some great work. We often make a vinegar acetum of it too as this can be very valuable added to baths or used on small wounds (she is a wound herb too, and not just skin wounds; wounds of every kind and to the emotions and psyche as well as the physical body). Selfheal balances the thyroid (actually she balances all sorts) and has even been shown to help with autoimmune conditions of the thyroid. She is very high in rosmarinic acid, a most potent antioxidant which helps with inflammation, allergic responses and improving immune function generally. She balances blood sugars and blood pressure. She has been shown to be effective against viral infections and even against the bacterial organism that causes TB. She is most plentiful when allowed to flourish, and she certainly does help us to heal ourselves. Glancing at Julie Bruton-Seal and Matthew Seal's book this evening, I noticed they say that the flower essence is good when you are ill and don't know where to turn for help; that really resonates. I could say much more but suffice to say when I was musing on what to write this evening and the mysteries of connecting with our plant kin (and with the rest of the natural world) she whispered the deepest mystery is being in love; like being and doing that in love. Well, that will heal pretty much anything. She's a sound friend for sure.

Vervain

Verbena officinalis Verbenaceae.

Many years ago, I was in Oxford walking past the Culpeper shop and spotted some fresh herb plants for sale. A little vervain plant drew me; it was not one I was familiar with. So, I bought it, took it home and had a wee nibble—it is very bitter! At first, she looks rather unassuming, but this plant has such a strength to her. Last year we gave the apprentices one each to sit with as a group, their first time trying this. They really got it, how she helps us hold ourselves up, erect but not taut, in our authentic self. Another group at a summer workshop tuned into a vervain plant in preparation for making a flower essence; even though some of them were quite unfamiliar with flower essences the results were impressive—I had left them listening to her under the care of Majella and when I came back there were five very calm people one of whom said that they felt like they could just stay there for the rest of the day; they spoke about the vitality they felt, how they felt very present and how the cares had just left them, they felt sovereign and truly in their own quiet power, vervain helps to regenerate nerve tissue. She is a wonderful bitter that tones the digestion and improves the absorption of food calm the nerves (especially if the hormones are out of balance, any hormones, not just the reproductive ones and restores the nervous system, releasing stress and anxiety). She works to balance the thyroid too. She helps move the circulation and cool fevers. She helps with headaches and migraines and can relieve insomnia. She is also an amazing immune tonic. She has traditionally been used as a smudge herb in Ireland and is native to this land, used to purify a space (or a person) and seen as a sacred plant (they all are really). She is thought of as a panacea, and a herb of peace, love, diplomacy and protection. She can stimulate the uterus so should not be used in pregnancy but can assist in labour. After childbirth, vervain will help both the restoring of the mother's vitality and also the establishment of a good milk flow to feed the baby.

Herb Robert

Geranium robertianum Geraniaceae.

About 7 years ago, we started to notice that herb robert plants were springing up all over the garden, and large healthy ones at that, they really seemed to be wanting some attention paid to them so I started to listen to the plants and then went over to Herbfeast in the UK where there were herb people from the US, France and lots of other people, and everyone was talking about this plant … and we started exchanging stories. Since then we have made aromatic waters, tinctures, vinegars, eaten it in salads, made infused oils for the skin and continue to get to know this puckish being more and more. It has much in common with other geraniums and also an essential character of their own. Some people like the aroma of this plant, others find it challenging. He is often overlooked as a weed but is a most incredible healer. One of the students used it to bring their blood pressure down; it also helps balance blood sugars whether they have a tendency to high or low and can reduce sugar cravings and can help balance blood fats too. He works with the Earth element, reducing worry, balancing our relationship with the Earth and our ability to receive and digest on all levels. He also helps to balance the solar plexus. This plant can help us to incarnate fully, properly into the person we were born to be; become free of the fear of walking our own journey and singing our own song. This is a plant that helps us to ground, that helps us to re-establish our boundaries if they have been disrupted. It helps us re-centre in our own authentic self and be able to hold this in how we relate to others; this is ideal for those who find themselves becoming ungrounded and lost in a relationship, helping us to maintain our separateness and ability to see the other. He can take a bit of time to get to know and may even insist on a formal introduction but once acquainted, he is a great teacher and messenger plant helping us to engage with other plant friends. The redness of the stems and the way it can help balance the blood pressure speak of how it helps us to circulate our heart energy through our own being and out into the world. The pink flowers definitely indicate this is a heart ally (most of this family are). The spear-like seed heads indicate that it is a heart warrior and heart protector plant; such plants help us to protect our hearts by reminding us to be fully incarnated and knowing who we are and therefore able to be open since we know what is us and what is other. The needle-like seed heads also speak of how this plant will help repair wounds (it is also a great wound herb physically) and can help with internal haemorrhage and also heavy menstrual bleeding. It has a good reputation as a plant that helps prevent mutagenesis and tumour formation. Last year Marion, a very gifted student, said that she felt it repaired the nerves; a little research and we discovered that it does indeed facilitate neurogenesis; very valuable as so many people are re-wiring their nervous systems. We have certainly had some wry and ironic jokes whilst harvesting the plentiful amounts that grow here to make different medicines.

Dandelion

Taraxacum officinale Asteraceae.

It is so wonderful when the dandelions wake up; they are one of the first flowers to feed the bees in the spring. Dandelion (*Taraxacum officinale*) is one of those common plants that is a most incredible healer others include nettles, plantain, elder, daisy (OK, there are quite a few), one of those plants that can be used to treat nearly anything. There are some plant medicine people who only work with one or maybe five plants, just a few; they do this as they know their ally/allies really well and know how to ask them for help for most things. Dandelion is a plant that will help for so many ailments. Although the plant is a diuretic (the leaves more so than the root) which helps flush excess fluid out of the body via the kidneys and remove excess acid from the body it is also so rich in potassium that it acts as a potassium supplement at the same time; most synthetic diuretics have to be taken alongside potassium as they deplete this precious mineral from the system. The diuretic action of dandelion gave rise to its French common name *Pis Enlit*. The leaves are delicious in salads; initially, one might find them a little bitter but adding some grated carrot or beetroot softens the bitterness and soon one gains a taste for those bitter greens and finds the desire for heavily sweet foods lessens; we made a rather lovely pesto from them with elderberry vinegar last year which improved if left to mature for a few hours—it was a pleasant surprise. The whole plant is also an amazing liver tonic and cleanser, increasing bile production and release with the root being considered stronger in this action. The roots can be used in stir fries or roasted to make a coffee substitute or decocted to treat the liver. Its action on the liver means it can be helpful in hormonal imbalances, skin conditions, arthritis and joint pain and many other conditions. Bitter herbs help to open and balance the heart, and Thomas Bartram says that dandelion root has an action similar to Beta blockers, lowering blood pressure and calming the system. Bitters also are wonderful nervines, possibly in part due to their action on the gut-brain—they are wonderful for improving low mood and anxiety as well. Dandelion increases bile flow, and bile is both antiseptic for our bowel and a laxative, so it cleans and clears the bowel too. Dandelion is a wonderful digestive tonic, toning the liver and the pancreas and also the root contains inulin which is a prebiotic. Dandelion can help with premenstrual symptoms, including water retention and mood disturbances and can also be useful in menopause. It is probably one of our local adaptogens. It can help with allergies and reducing catarrh by toning the digestion. The petals can be added to salads for their colour and wee bit of flavour; we tried making syrup from them, we really tried, but it came out very insipid. The sap from the flower stems can be used to treat warts and verrucae. The leaf is jagged and gives the plant its name: dandelion is a corruption of the French for lion's teeth. The leaves help to clear fear from the heart and rain it out through the kidneys—this process can increase urination substantially increasing the need for fluid and salt intake initially. The root clears anger and other emotions that have stagnated in the liver and the bowel; the cleaning and tonifying action on the liver and pancreas and digestive system can help us to absorb and process emotions and emotional backlogs. Sometimes when given to people who are rather meek, who have suppressed their anger and been nice and quiet all their lives, they find that they are speaking up for themselves and standing up for themselves rather more strongly. In other words, dandelion helps us to recover our lion's heart (teeth and all), our courage and our passion. With that vibrant yellow colour of the flowers, it is most assuredly a plant of the sun and the solar plexus. There are many other things the dandelion can help with; this plant is most definitely not a common weed; it is a noble and totally underrated food and medicine which deserves a lot more respect. And by the way, there are a couple of hundred subspecies of dandelion.

Mints

The mints are a group that continually surprise me with more and more learnings about their medicine. They are wonderful for clearing our thoughts when they have been fuzzed by too much external input and also for clearing our energy field—a good bunch for the times we live in, I guess. The mints are all perennials and spread by root runners so can take over a bit, hence the pots. Some are cultivars, some are species, and the peppermint is a hybrid.

We have several kinds of mint here:

- Peppermint (a hybrid of *Mentha aquatica* and *Mentha spicata*), *Mentha x piperita*. True peppermint must be raised from cuttings (or by cross-pollinating the two parent species), as it is a hybrid it cannot be raised from seed.
- Spearmint (*Mentha spicate*).
- Green mint (*Mentha viridis*).
- Water mint (Mentha aquatica).
- The tiny Corsican mint (*Mentha requenii*), which looks almost like a tiny moss and has flowers just a couple of mm across.
- The *eau de cologne* mint.

Mints are wonderful used fresh and can be harvested for drying just before the flowers open. They must be dried carefully to conserve aromatic element. The name comes from a Greek legend about Menthe who was a nymph who attracted the lustful eye of Zeus and was turned into a plant to protect her chastity. Peppermint is considered to be very clearing to the mind and energy field. It helps the clarity of thinking but is also good if one feels overloaded with other peoples' energy or ideas. It can also help if one finds other people draining to one's energy. It is another of the herbs that help restore vagal tone (hence its use in smelling salts) and so can relax without sedating. It is both pungent and cooling. Some authors feel that peppermint is not suitable for children under 5, and its oil is not suitable for children under 5 according to some authors, whilst other authors state that it should not be used for children under 12 years of age.

However, other mints are safe for all ages. The mints have a huge range of actions; relaxing spasms, calming the digestion, reducing wind, helping to sweat, reducing fever, encouraging bile production, preventing nausea and vomiting, toning the liver, stimulating or maybe balancing the nervous system, improving circulation to the head and therefore the ability to think. They are also decongestant and expectorant and antiviral against colds but also shingles and colds sores. Peppermint constricts the blood vessels. All the mints are anti-inflammatory, and topically they reduce itching and are antiseptic and antifungal as well as being analgesic and insect repellent. They have effects on the hormonal system, reducing heavy menstrual bleeding in some cases, reducing milk production when weaning a baby and reducing androgen production.

Mints are well known for benefiting the digestion, hence after dinner mints and liqueurs. They can help with gripping wind, diarrhoea, nausea and vomiting. They also help with IBS, travel sickness and gastroenteritis.

They are used to treat the common cold, flus and fevers; as an infusion, often combined with elderflower and yarrow, but they well alone too. They can help with heavy and painful periods and work on the ovaries to help irregular and infrequent periods.

Mints help with headaches and migraines, especially linked to digestive weakness. They also help with rhinitis and sinusitis, by reducing mucus.

They also help with low blood pressure, probably by working on vagal balance. In addition, they promote clear thinking, relieve apathy, nervous palpitations and vertigo Topically—one can use the infusion or diluted essential oil to relieve the pain of bruises, sciatica, shingles or neuralgia and also itching of eczema, herpes, and urticaria. They are also used as a repellent for gnats, mosquitoes, lice, scabies, rats and ants. Spearmint tea seems to reduce the number of androgens produced. This can reduce libido in men, and can reduce hirsutism in women with polycystic ovaries.

Bay

Laurus nobilis Lauraceae.

We make bay and ash aromatic water every year because it is so wonderful; my friend Susy makes an acetum of the two and uses it when driving a long distance and pronounces it more effective than the Red Bull she used to use for focus and energy on long trips. It is a wonderful remedy, combining the guardian energy of the bay tree with the energy of the ash which helps us to be whom we feel we are, and move into integrity and flexibility; the combination feels like it brings focus and boundaries and a wonderful sense of being grounded, empowered and strong in ourselves. It helped bring me back to life a couple of years ago. Bay is not native but is a guardian tree and watches as the guardian of a place, of the home, which is perhaps one of the reasons so many have this tree in their garden. It is also a wonderful stimulating nervine and stimulates the digestion. It is strongly antimicrobial and has been used for centuries as a cooking herb that brings warmth to our food but also protects us against infection. The prunings can be dried and used as a smudge or added to winter fires to clear space and keep the air sweet and free of bugs. It makes a wonderful addition to rich stews, tomato sauces and soups. I find our bay tree to be a steadying and steadfast friend. Bay is also wonderful for the mind—the term Laureate comes from this plant, and traditionally champions and scholars were crowned with a wreath of laurel leaves. There is much more to learn from this noble tree. Bay has also been shown to lower blood sugars, and blood fats so is a valuable treatment for late-onset diabetes or pre-diabetic tendencies and for cholesterol. Bay is well known as a hair tonic and for treating skin infections due to its antifungal and antimicrobial actions. It is also used as an udder wash by vets and farmers.

Horseradish

Amoracia rusticana Brassicaceae.

From a young age, I loved the taste and pungency of this herb, and I am continually astonished at how far-reaching its healing powers are. Before wasabi became such a popular condiment in this part of the world, horseradish sauce was a staple. In fact, most of the wasabi sauces sold here are primarily made from horseradish and mustard with just a little of the wasabi root to give that green colour and its own inimitable character.

Horseradish is thought to be a native of southern Russia but has been naturalised here for a very long time; it prefers damp conditions but grows happily on field margins, waste ground and at the coast. It is easy to cultivate from root slips; if growing for roots, then a deep dug well-manured trench will give strong straight roots, easy to harvest. The long, lanceolate leaves can be used as well as the roots and both parts of the plant are extremely pungent, one of our native heating herbs. The dried root loses some of its potency but is still an effective remedy and food.

Fresh root tea is be infused in warm water (not hot, as too much heat converts isothiocyanates to detrimental constituents).

Horseradish can have a tendency to take over in the garden if not regularly harvested and divided, but there are many interesting foods and great medicines to prepare from it. It is harvested in the spring or autumn for highest activity but can be harvested anytime.

Horseradish sauce, a traditional accompaniment for beef but also good with mackerel and a lot of other foods. The leaves can be used to make a wasabi-like sauce—for this we combine leaves, roots, some Dijon mustard and sometimes some onion, chopping them all finely or grinding them in a Nutri bullet. We also use horseradish in our fire cider or dragon's brew (I prefer the latter name). Another favourite is horseradish mayonnaise. We blend a few horseradish leaves, some grated root, a little red onion and a dash of vinegar or lemon juice into vegan mayonnaise and use this as an accompaniment to potato cakes and bean burgers. The sauce helps to warm and stimulate our digestion.

It's pungency, and therapeutic properties, are mainly due to Mustard oil glycosides, including sinigrin which is strongly antibacterial, especially for lungs and urinary tract, warming, reduce thyroid activity, digestive regulator and cleanser. It also contains resin, vitamin C, vitamin B, and asparagine which is diuretic.

The fresh, grated root is used to treat hay fever; one takes a level teaspoon of the grated root and chews it, inducing an eye-watering, nose stinging effect that also gets the nose running thoroughly. It is something of a heroic treatment but very effective. I tried it one summer when an unusually bad bout of hay fever was impeding my ability to study, and the results of one treatment were miraculous.

A syrup is sometimes prepared by covering the freshly grated root with sugar (or apple juice concentrate here as sugar is just too sweet for our taste) and leaving it to steep at room temperature overnight. This is then stored in the fridge for use in asthma, bronchitis and catarrh (grated turnip can be substituted and has a milder action).

Horseradish is used to stimulate the appetite and the digestive system, although too much can cause digestive cramps or be emetic. It sterilises the stomach contents and stimulates the production of acid and enzymes, probably a reflex from irritation of gut and mouth.

It is stimulating in general due to its effect on the circulation, increasing sweating and expectorating mucus, and has rubefacient effect when applied topically. Along with this, it is a diuretic, and so these combined actions make it an excellent cleansing and detoxifying ally.

It is used externally in poultices or liniments for gout, rheumatism, joint pain and stiff muscles and can also be used to affect deeper organs and tissues by reflex action through the dermatomes apply over kidney, liver and spleen, heart/lungs to increase function. For bronchial treatment, apply over the chest and around the face to inhale. It increases the blood flow to the tissues, and this speeds up healing time. However, it can cause blisters if applied for too long or in too high a concentration but applying a layer over oil under the poultice and limiting application time will prevent this happening. The active constituents are absorbed through the gut wall or skin and attach to red blood cells in the blood. They are then excreted from blood via kidneys and lungs.

Horseradish inhibits the flu virus. It is an effective disinfectant for wounds and used to prepare poultice for slow healing wounds. It increases regeneration of tissues and therefore is good for ulcerous wounds (high in vitamin C). It also checks the growth of many pathogenic bacteria and so keeps wounds clean whilst healing.

As a diuretic horseradish can be used to treat oedema or kidney stones and increases micturation (possibly diuretic) which increases uric acid secretion. Horseradish is a possible pancreatic remedy and can overcome risks of chronic high or low blood sugar levels. It stops the secretion of thyroid hormones and induces goitre in those susceptible so should be avoided in hypothyroidism, myxoedema and goitre, but it is useful in treating overactive thyroid.

Also, avoid with gastritis and severe high blood pressure.

Bilberry, huckleberry, whortleberry, hurtleberry, blueberry, frauchan

Vaccinium myrtillus Ericaceae.

Bilberry and blueberry have become key allies over the last while. I had always valued bilberry for its support to the eyes helping us with our night vision; bilberry jam was given to pilots in World War II to help them see in the dark. Bilberry is one of our native adaptogens, very similar in some ways to shisandra. One day, I was out in the garden musing on what the energetics of bilberry and blueberry were so I started listening to the plants here and asked them what they do on that level, and the reply was: help you see in the dark. I was about to say that I know that is what they do physically when I had a double or triple aha moment; they help us to see in the long dark night of the soul too, and secondly that the physical effects describe the energetic effects and thirdly that a significant encounter with bilberries in the wild was on a ritual walk with a friend and my kids after my father had died. A few months after the conversation with the plants in the garden, the same friend (who happens to be a psychologist) sent me a paper about blueberry and its value in treating PTSD; this is in part due to the fact that the proantho-cyanidins slot into our endocannabinoid receptors in a way that neither stimulates nor calms them, just makes them feel neutral, and this is of great help for those with both PTSD and complex trauma symptoms; we see a lot of people displaying these symptoms these days in no small part due to the pathological society we live in which marginalises and traumatises many people who have been told to get over it and fit in.

The fact that the leaves (and berries, especially in Scandinavia and Russia) are used to balance blood sugars, treat diabetes and therefore work on the solar plexus is indicative of the fact that the plant helps us to digest the information that comes in at those times of soul searching and intensive interior work. The anthocyanins that repair tissues and reduce inflammation show how it protects and repairs our tissues but also help us with stressful overloads of energetic information and the plant also helps to repair the circulation, helps keep our energy moving and circulating when we feel like pulling in and closing down. The plant also helps prevent haemorrhaging of our energy.

In Ireland, bilberries were regularly mentioned as a favourite wild food in early monastic poetry. They were traditionally collected at Lughnasadh (1st August) or Lammas (first Sunday in August). Fraughan Sunday was a day of festivities before the harvest began and was also a traditional day for courtship. The taste of the berries is sweet, and slightly sour due to the presence of oligomeric proanthocyanins, fruit acids, phenolic acids, vitamin B_1, C and carotene. The pectin contributes to the sweetness, and flavonoids give some bitterness and tannins give a little dryness to the taste.

Bilberry is a circulatory tonic and vasodilator which improves capillary function and increases capillary strength and reduces permeability. It is therefore used to treat petechiae, easy bruising and nosebleeds. It heals inflammation in the circulatory system and is a phlebotonic used to treat varicose veins, piles, Raynaud's and inter-mittent claudication. Its action on the capillaries makes it a valuable treatment for some forms of menorrhagia and also for primary dysmen-orrhoea. I remember giving it to one young woman with Raynaud's who had not mentioned her painful, heavy periods for which she regularly took Ponstan. After three weeks on the herbs, she returned and reported that not only was her circulation much improved but also her period was much more manageable which she viewed as quite remarkable since she had forgotten to mention that they were problematic. The anti-inflammatory properties probably also help here. In addition, as a circulatory tonic bilberry can help relieve fluid retention, pain, pins and needles, paraesthesia, migraine and cramps caused by impaired peripheral blood flow.

As already mentioned, bilberry is used to treat eye problems associated with reduced blood flow to the area especially in high blood pressure and diabetes; these include simple glaucoma, retinitis, and it corrects visual fatigue by replenishing retina purple as well as helping to prevent cataract formation.

Along with other anthocyanin-rich berries such as hawthorn, elderberries and rosehips, bilberry stabilises collagen and helps to repair it. This means these fruits can help repair blood vessels and also the GIT lining, reducing inflammation in the gut and therefore throughout the body. It can be used both as a mild laxative or to treat diarrhoea; it's action on the bowel being balancing or amphoteric.

It is a mild antibacterial and can help treat urinary tract infections; its cousin cranberry has been shown to prevent bacteria adhering to the bladder wall due to the presence of hyaluronic acid.

As a food bilberries and blueberries are absolutely amazing to use in smoothies, syrups, vinegars, pies, and muffins. We never manage to bring enough home from our forages to make much with, they all get eaten on the way (and they turn your tongue the most interesting shade of blue). When one picks them, one appreciates the relatively high price of them bought in tincture and dried berries—it takes a lot of work, but the wonderful Scandinavian berry combs do help.

Oats

Avena sativa Graminaceae.

Oats are such an amazing food-medicine. The ripe seeds contain starch, protein, fats, including tocopherol (vitamin E), prolamines—avenins, C-glycosyl flavones, minerals, particularly silica and calcium, vitamins, especially B group, saponins, alkaloids and sterols and can be used in countless ways. Our current favourites are using oat groats in stews and soups in a similar way to how pearly barley is used and also laverbread cake which is like vegan white pudding with the added benefit of seaweed in it. Oats have a lovely nourishing flavour—sweet, mealy and neutral in temperature.

Oat grass can be juiced in the same way as wheatgrass, and the flowering tops or oat straw make a most splendid nerve tonic which is very valuable for nervous teenage students, nervous students of any age, breastfeeding mothers and those in their senior years, actually for anyone who needs their nervous system replenishing and nourishing and the fact that it is neither cooling nor heating makes it a panacea for all people in my view.

All parts of the oat plant are a nerve tonic par excellence; antidepressive, thymoleptic and trophorestorative. And suitable for treating depression, melancholia, menopausal neurasthenia, general debility, especially from chronic pain or insomnia and convalescence.

The oat seed is a valuable cardiac tonic being high in calcium and is also helpful in treating hyperlipidaemia due to the soft fibre it contains (the bran is especially helpful). The soft fibre is also helpful for irritable bowel symptoms and for constipation. Oats are a nutritive tonic food which help to improve stamina and muscle function and help to build bone and teeth, especially in children.

Oats can also be used topically as an emollient. They make a valuable skin cleanser and softener for those who are sensitive to detergents and soap. Place fine oatmeal in a muslin bag and use as a substitute for soap. This is soothing for eczema and itchy skin and can be complemented by adding the muslin bag of oatmeal into the bath. Fine oatmeal can be used to make purifying face packs for acne and congested skin or as a base for a poultice to draw out congestion from the skin.

Orange blossom

Citrus aurantium flos Rutaceae.

I originally came across orange blossom medicine in the form of neroli essential oil during my aromatherapy training; it is a most beautiful aroma but very expensive, so I reserved it for special treatments and often used petitgrain, the oil from the leaves and immature fruit, as a substitute. I then discovered the hydrosol or aromatic water and loved working with this but still mainly for treating the skin.

Then, about 10 years ago, Joe Nasr introduced me to his aromatic water and mentioned how it was used like rescue remedy in his native

Lebanon; coincidentally, I was widening my explorations of Middle Eastern cooking and noticed that orange blossom water is an ingredient widely used in several recipes.

In the last decade, orange blossom aromatic water has become a mainstay of our pharmacy. We find it useful as a digestive tonic due to its action on the liver and pancreas; it may also be useful for diabetes. It is used for diarrhoea and digestive upsets, especially when nervous in origin since it is also neurotonic. Combined with its antispasmodic action, it can be valuable in the treatment of IBS and spastic colon.

It is also a most amazing nervine and treatment for trauma, but acute and chronic, or for PTSD and complex trauma. For example, one day a student arrived having severely scalded her foot by dropping a glass teapot on it. Although she had treated the scald, she was still very shaken and in pain. A 10 ml dose of orange blossom water had her feeling calm within 10 minutes. Another day a student arrived very shaken after a traumatic telephone conversation with a work colleague, and again the single dose of the aromatic water calmed her down within a few minutes.

I have given doses to patients who have come for myofascial unwinding to clear traumas, and it really helps the work to proceed more easily; it helps the trauma leave the body without having to revisit it. For this reason, I often include it in prescriptions for those working on trauma issues or symptoms made worse by complex trauma. I also include it in pain mixtures since it really does help relieve nerve pain and to harmonise the other herbs together.

It is known to lower high blood pressure but I find it amphoteric, raising low blood pressure to a healthier level, especially if it drops as part of a vasovagal response. Orange blossom water seems to balance the vagal tone, especially if it is in an overly sympathetic mode. It is an immediately calming medicine and also helps lift low mood, and treat anxiety and nervousness and even lack of confidence.

Topically, it is cytophylatic (promotes healthy skin growth) especially if the skin is dry and sensitive. It is a very safe remedy which can be used throughout pregnancy.

Wood betony

Stachys officinalis, *Stachys betonica* Lamiaceae/Labiatae.

When we started the student training clinics about 10 years ago, we were using about half a litre of *Stachys* a year in the dispensary;

it had somehow fallen under the radar and out of use. Within a couple of months though it had caught the students' attention and we were getting through a half litre per month. It remains a favourite herb, especially as a local adaptogen that supports the adrenals and vagal balance.

According to Culpeper, Antonius Musa, physician to Emperor Augustus, listed 47 uses of betony, including protection from snakes and from evil. An Italian saying from fourteenth-century Italy is 'May you have more virtue than betony'. In the Middle Ages, it was cultivated in monastic gardens and graveyards to protect against witchcraft and would be worn as an amulet around the neck or placed under the pillow for protection. It was regarded as a panacea for all ills.

The herb is cool, drying, bitter and sweet and the leaves emit a wonderful aroma when crushed in the hand.

The plant contains alkaloids, including stachydrine and betonicine, betaine, choline, tannins. The alkaloids make it unsuitable for use during pregnancy.

The common name betony derives from Gaelic for good head because so much of its medicine helps heal the head. It is helpful in the treatment of headaches and migraine, recovery from head injuries, facial pain, sinus headaches and congestion, nosebleeds and toothache.

It also helps calm an overactive mind and general overactivity, insomnia caused by a racing mind, gathers scattered thoughts, relieves anxiety, irritability, depression. It improves concentration and poor memory and is good for nervous tension, including premenstrual tension and is good for nervous exhaustion since it is a general nerve tonic improving nerve function. It helps us to face the fears and evils in our own minds and so is useful for withdrawal from addictive drugs, including prescribed medications. It can help alleviate feelings of spaciness and unconnectedness. It also balances the solar plexus, grounds us and connects us to the Earth.

Much of this nervine action is due to it being an aromatic bitter which also gives it many of its digestive tonic properties. Betony tones the liver, gallbladder and digestion and is soothing for IBS, gastritis, inflammation and tension in the bowel. It is also good for those who are underweight as it stimulates the appetite if this has been absent and also calms the adrenals.

It is a tonic for older people or in convalescence from a long illness as a general tonic, increasing strength mentally, physically and spiritually; or those who feel unwell without any recognisable cause.

It is very effective in prolapse of the uterus and other organs, especially when combined with *Astragalus*. One remarkable result of this combination, when used on a young woman with a prolapsed cervix, was that after two weeks on the formula when she went to her physiotherapist who had inserted a cervical support ring and was treating her regularly was told by the therapist that her cervix had reverted to normal. Although it should not be used in pregnancy, it can help during a weak labour and also can reduce excessive menstruation.

Betony (and some of the other members of the *Stachys* genus) may be used externally in an ointment for bruises, sprains, strains, varicose veins, and haemorrhoids. A poultice can be prepared from the fresh herb to treat bruises and wounds. An infusion can be used to bathe leg ulcers and infected wounds or used as a mouthwash for mouth ulcers, sore gums and sore throats.

The tea is pleasant to drink and can be used for indigestion, headache, poor circulation, muscular tension, nightmares, sinus congestion, watery and irritated eyes, head colds, chills and fevers and insomnia. It is a cleansing herb used in arthritis and toxic conditions. We have also found it to be a pleasant-smelling smudge herb that helps to ground us and to clear the air of any bad humours.

NOTES

It was nearly impossible to choose which 25 allies to include here, and so the end note is a list of those whom I wish to acknowledge for the amazing work they do and for all the wonderful teachings they have given me and for being such generous friends.

Agrimony, alexanders, alkanet, allspice, *Anemone pulsatilla*, arrowroot, asparagus, *Asparagus racemosa*, *Astragalus*, barberry, basil, bear's breeches, beech, birch, blackcurrant, bog bean, borage, bramble, broad bean, bugle, butcher's broom, cabbage, cardamom, centuary, chamomile, chervil, chickweed, chicory, chilli, *Cistus landifer*, cleavers, clove pink, *Codonopsis*, coltsfoot, cowslip, coriander, couchgrass, Cuban Oregano, cumin, curled dock, cypress, dahlias, dill, enchanter's nightshade, evening primrose, fat hen, fennel, fenugreek, feverfew, flaxseed, foxglove, ginger, ginkgo, globe artichoke, *Grindelia*, guelder rose, hairy bittercress, hazel, hebe, heartsease, holly, honeysuckle, hops, houttuynia, hydrangea, hyssop, immortelle, ivy, jasmine, Jerusalem artichoke, juniper, kalonji, lady's mantle, lady's smock, lamb's ear, lamb's lettuce, lavender, lemon, lemon balm, lemon *Verbena*, lilac, lovage, lungwort, maize, marsh cudweed, meadowsweet, miner's lettuce, mugwort, mullein, musk mallow, mustard, *Myrica*, myrtle, *Nasturtium*, nectarine, neem, olive, orange, oregano, oxeye daisy, parsley, paeony, paprika, peace lily, pear, pepper, pine, pineapple sage, poached egg plant, potato, purslane, Rapunzel, red clover, rocket, rose geranium, rosebay willowherb, rue, Saint John's wort, sage, salad burnet, sanicle, *Schisandra*, skullcap, sneezewort, soapwort, sorrel, sow thistle, sphagnum moss, speedwell, spider plant, spirea, spruce, strawberry, sweet cicely, sweet violet, sweet woodruff, tarragon, teasel, thyme, tulsi, turmeric, viper's bugloss, white horehound, wild celery, wild cherry, willow, witch hazel, withania, woad, wood avens, wormwood, yellow pimpernel, yellow toadflax, yarrow, yew, zallouh, *Zanthoxylum*, the mushroom folk, the seaweed people, the lichens and last but not least the tree ferns.

And those I am looking forward to deepening my friendships with such as gorse, heather, purple loosestrife, and so many more.

BIBLIOGRAPHY

Abrams, David, *The Spell of the Sensuous* (New York, NY: Vintage Books, 1996).

Ackerman, Dian, *A Natural History of the Senses* (London: Chapmans, 1990).

Barker, Julian, *The Medicinal Flora of Britain And North-western Europe* (West Wickham, 2001).

Bartram, Thomas, *Encyclopaedia of Herbal Medicine* (Dorset: Grace Publishers, 1996).

Blamey, Marjorie, Richard Sidney, Richmond Fitter, Alastair H Fitter, *Wild Flowers of Britain and Ireland* (London: A&C Publishers, 2003).

Bown, Deni, *The Royal Horticultural Society Encylopedia of Herbs and Their Uses* (London: BCA, 1995).

Brooke, Elizabeth, *A Woman's Book of Herbs* (London: Aeon Books Ltd, 2018).

Bruneton, Jean, *Pharmacognosy, Phytochemistry, Medicinal Plants* (Andover: Intercept limited, 1995).

Bruton-Seal, Julie and Matthew Seal, *Hedgerow Medicine* (Ludlow: Merlin Unwin, 2008).

Bruton-Seal, Julie and Matthew Seal, *Wayside Medicine* (Ludlow: Merlin Unwin, 2017).

Burgess, Yvonne, *The Myth of Progress* (Glasgow: Wild Goose Publications, 1996).

Caddy, Rosemary, *Essential Oils in Colour* (Horsley: Amberwood Publishing, 1997).

Cech, Richo, *The Medicinal Herb Grower* (Williams, OR: Horizon Herbs, 2009).

Cecho, Richo, *Making Plant Medicines* (Williams, OR: Horizon Herbs, 2000).

Chevalier, Andrew, *Encyclopaedia of Herbal Medicine* (London: Dorling Kindersley, 2016).

Childre, Doc and Howard Martin, with Donna Beech, *The Heart Math Solution* (New York: Harper Collins, 2000).

Clarke, Sue, *Essential Chemistry for Safe Aromatherapy* (London: Churchill Livingstone, 2002).

Cohen, Ed, *A Body Worth Defending* (Durham: Duke University Press, 2009).

de Baircali Levy, Juliette, *Common Herbs of Natural Health* (Woodstock: Ash Tree Publishing, 1997).

Devlin, Zoe, *Irish Wildflowers* (Cork: The Collins Press, 2014).

Eisler, Rian, *The Chalice and the Blade* (San Francisco, CA: Harper & Row, 1988).

Estés, Clarissa Pinkoka, *Women Who Run with the Wolves* (New York, NY: Ballantine Books, Random House, 1995).

Frederici, Silvia, *Caliban and the Witch* (New York, NY: Autonomedia, 2004).

Frederici, Silvia, *Re-enchanting the World* (Oakland, CA: PM Press, 2019).

Green, James, *The Herbal Medicine Maker's Handbook; A Home Manual* (Berkeley, CA: The Crossing Press, 2000).

Grenham, Sue, Gerard Clarke, John F. Cryan and Timothy G. Dinan. Brain–gut–microbe communication in health and disease. *Frontiers in Physiology* 2011; 2: 94.

Grieve, Maud, *A Modern Herbal* (London: Penguin Books, 1988).

Griggs, Barbara, *New Green Pharmacy* (London: Ebury Press Random House, 1997).

Hatfield, Gabrielle and David Allen, *Medicinal Plants in Folk Tradition* (Cambridge: Timber Press, 2004).

Hatfield, Gabrielle, *Hatfield's Herbal* (London: Penguin, 2007).

Hatfield, Gabrielle, *Memory, Wisdom and Healing* (Stroud: Sutton Publishing, 1999).

Hedley, Christopher and Non Shaw, *Herbal Remedies* (Bath: Paragon, 2002).

Heinrich, Michael et al., *Fundamentals of Pharmacognosy and Phytotherapy* (London: Churchill Livingstone, 2004).

Hughes, Nathaniel, *Weeds in The Heart* (London: Aeon Books and Quintessence Press, 2018).

Hyams, Roger and Richard Pankhurst, *Plants and Their Names* (Oxford: The Oxford University Press, 1995).

Jarmey, Chris, *The Concise Book of Muscles* (Chichester: Lotus Press, 2003).

Juhan, Deane, *Job's Body* (Barrytown, NY: Barrytown/Station Hill Press, 2003).

Kindred, Glennie, *Earth Wisdom* (London: Hay House, 2005).

Kindred, Glennie, *Letting in the Wild Edges* (East Meon: Permanent Publications, 2013).

Kress, Henriette, *Practical Herbs 1+2 and Practical Herb Cards* (Helsinki: Yrtit ja yrttiterpia Henriette Kress, 2013, 2013, 2017).

Leggett, Daverick, *Recipes for Self Healing* (Totnes: Meridian Press, 1999).

Lipton, Bruce, *Biology of Belief* (London: Hay House, 2008).

Mabey, Richard, *Flora Britannica* (London: Chatto & Windus, 1997).

Mabey, Richard, *Weeds* (London: Profile Books, 2010).

Mac Coitir, Niall, *Irish Wild Plants* (Cork: Collins Press, 2006).

Mac Coitir, Niall, *Irish Trees* (Cork: Collins Press, 2003).

Matthews, Caitlin and John Matthews, *Encyclopedia of Celtic Wisdom* (London: Rider Books, 2001).

Mauseth, James, Botany, *An Introduction to Plant Biology* (Toronto: Jones and Bartlett, 1998).

Mc Garry, Gina, *Brighid's Healing* (Sutton Mallet, Green Magic Publishing, 2005).

McGilchrist, Iain, The *Master and his Emissary* (New Haven, CT: Yale University Press, 2010).

McVicar, Jekka, *Jekka's Complete Herb Book* (London: Kyle Cathie, 1997).

Milne, Hugh, *The Heart of Listening* (Berkeley, CA: North Atlantic Books, 1995).

Pengelly, Andrew, *The Constituents of Medicinal Plants* (Merriwa: Sunflower Herbals, 1996).

Pert, Candace, *Molecules of Emotion* (New York, NY: Simon & Shuster, 1999).

Phillips, Roger, *Wild Food* (London: Pan Macmillan, 1983).

Phillips, Roger, and Nicky Foy, *Herbs* (London: Pan Books, 1992).

Pole, Sebastian, *Ayurvedic Medicine* (London: Churchill Livingstone, 2006).

Reichstein, Gail, *Chinese Medicine in Everyday Life* (New York, NY: Kodansha America, Inc, 1998).

Reynolds, Mary, *The Garden Awakening* (Cambridge: Green Books, 2016)

Reynolds Thompson, Mary, *Reclaiming the Wild Soul* (Ashland, OR: White Cloud Press, 2014)

Scott, Tommy Lee, *Invasive Plant Medicine* (Rochester, VT: Healing Arts Press, 2010)

Snyder, Gary, *The Practice of the Wild* (Berkeley, CA: Counterpoint, 2010).

Tobyn, Graeme, *Culpeper's Herbal Practice of Western Holistic Medicine* (Shaftesbury: Element Books, 1997).

Wall Kimmerer, Robin, *Braiding Sweetgrass* (Minneapolis, MN: Milkweed Editions, 2013).

Wolfe, Naomi, *Vagina A New Biography* (London: Virago Press, 2012).

INDEX